Ask Your Doctor, Ask Yourself

ASK YOUR DOCTOR ASK YOURSELF

Annette Thornhill

Para Research
Gloucester
Massachusetts

Ask Your Doctor, Ask Yourself
by Annette Thornhill

Copyright © 1986 Annette Thornhill
Cover design copyright © 1986 Para Research, Inc.

Library of Congress Card Number: 84-062728
International Standard Book Number: 0-914918-67-2

Typeset in 11 pt. Caslon on Compugraphic MCS/8400
Printed by Alpine Press, Inc. on 55-pound SRT II Paper
Edited by Emily McKeigue and Camilla Ayers
Cover design by Bob Boeberitz
Cover illustration by Tom Speck
Typeset by Patrice Banks and Camilla Ayers
160 pages

Published by Para Research, Inc.
85 Eastern Avenue
Gloucester, Massachusetts 01930

Manufactured in the United States of America

First Printing, April 1986, 3,000 copies

Contents

Author's Note

I have presented medical information as clearly and concisely as possible, but assume no responsibility for consequences resulting from suggestions, preparations, or therapies discussed. Nothing in this book is intended to take the place of traditional, legitimate, and licensed medical care. Self-treatment can be dangerous, and you are therefore encouraged to consult your doctor.

Publisher's Note

The publisher is pleased to be able to provide the author an opportunity to share with the public the thoughts and discussions embodied in this book. The reader should understand, however, that the publisher in no way endorses, recommends, or advocates any of the opinions offered or the suggestions, preparations, or therapies discussed. The publisher stresses the grave dangers inherent in any medical diagnosis or treatment which is not closely supervised by a competent, licensed doctor. This book is not intended to replace, or to be an alternative to such closely supervised diagnosis and treatment.

Acknowledgments

My thanks and gratitude go to the people who have helped me prepare the material for this book. Of necessity, they must remain anonymous, due to their profession and the controversial nature of the material herein contained.

My special gratitude to Dr. Emil K. Schandl of Dania, Florida, in particular, for the time and attention he gave me, in spite of his crowded schedule.

Introduction

The medical profession, because of its control over life-and-death matters, has an awesome and formidable power. We have granted doctors this power, for we have been assured they have the education and experience to provide us with the diagnoses and treatment we need.

However, it is long overdue for us as patients to reexamine the authority we have relinquished to the medical profession. As medical consumers, we must learn to participate more fully in our health care. We must learn where to find health resources, how to confirm diagnoses and how to make sound personal medical judgments.

The information in this book, gathered during the years I served as a medical librarian, was derived from research as well as discussions with reliable and responsible medical authorities. The book represents an attempt to bring together, in simple terms, information which will help those who are ready for greater involvement in their own health care.

A beginning must be made by you and by me—the ordinary people. We must *examine* the legislation passed by our elected representatives. In many cases, legislators have enacted into law restrictions which prevent many of us from helping ourselves and each other. For example:

> —In most states, you cannot independently use a laboratory and have the test results sent directly to you. Legislation requires that the tests be authorized by your doctor and that the results be sent directly to the physician. If you would like a copy of the results, it must come from the doctor's office.

> —In California it is illegal for the Licensing Commission for the medical profession to review a doctor's previous record in health care. The courts there have included those who discuss and advise on obesity or nervousness among those who need a license "to practice medicine."

> —In many states medical licensing laws have been framed in such broad language that, if strictly enforced, they would exclude husbands and lovers from the delivery room; unlicensed people would no longer be able to care for chronically ill family members; and scientists doing research on diseases could be charged with practicing medicine without a license.

Such restrictions serve to protect doctors, giving them sole jurisdiction over definitions such as "minimal brain dysfunction," and "learning disability."[1] They may also determine whether your pain is "real" or not and who shall or shall not be treated.[2]

We need these rights returned to us, so that we may have greater autonomy over our own health care, and the care of people dear to us. This may take some time. In the meantime, we can move toward that goal by working together, by using each other's experiences and by employing alternative therapies.

Learning about the tests you may do yourself before you go to the doctor will help you to confirm diagnoses.

In addition to checking a diagnosis, you should learn more than you are likely to be told about the medication you are ordered to take. You should learn about alternative forms of therapy if standard medicine does not solve your problems.

In this book I have tried to meet the needs of the people who came to me at the medical library and asked for help. They were never turned away, and I realized how anxious they were for answers that were being withheld, or for an alternate diagnosis their doctor had not considered. They were ready to do the leg work and the head work to find the answers.

If this book encourages you to make greater efforts toward finding and maintaining your own good health, communicating with your doctor, and actively participating in arriving at diagnoses and treatment, I will have attained my goal.

To those who assured me there were many people who would be grateful for such information, I dedicate this book.

NOTES

1. Ivan Illich, *Medical Nemesis*, p. 169.
2. Ibid., p. 47.

. . .each is the proper guardian of his own health, whether bodily, or mental and spiritual. . .

—John Stuart Mill

1

Tests You Can
Do Yourself

Let me relate an experience that might strike a familiar chord with
many people.

The pain was so severe that sweat collected on my forehead. In the
morning it was almost impossible for me to awaken and prepare the children
for school. I could barely coordinate arms, legs and body.

The doctor said I had arthritis and should begin treatment immediately.
First there was a weekly series of injections that nauseated me. Nothing
seemed to decrease the pain or the difficulty of making my limbs respond
to their cues. Discouraged, I insisted that some other remedy be considered,
and then I was started on a series of treatments that involved placing a wet
canvas bag on a plastic dish. The back of my left hand was placed against
the bag, giving as much contact as possible, while an electrode was pressed
against the palm of my right hand. After the treatment, black lines appeared
in my palm that did not disappear for a week—by which time I was due

for another treatment. After several weeks, I became discouraged with the lack of improvement, the expense of the visits and the trips to the office.

I was easily persuaded to change my physician, even though the first doctor was considered an authority on the treatment of arthritis. Test followed test in the office of the new doctor. Finally he told me I had never had arthritis and probably never would, judging by the structure and condition of my body. I had a condition known as hypothyroidism—and had spent hundreds of dollars I could ill afford, and a year and a half with a doctor who did not understand my condition.

Evidently it was time for me to stop believing in the infallibility of doctors and to start learning some self-care techniques for myself.

Over a period of time I discovered there were tests I could do myself with kits or materials purchased over the counter. Many pharmaceutical companies are making it possible for people to do some of their own testing either before they go to a doctor, or after a doctor's examination or laboratory testing to confirm the results. The idea of a "second opinion" has permeated the consciousness of many people who have misgivings about medical care in general, and the accuracy of test results in particular. The second opinion in a lot of cases can be your own.

The tests suggested here are not the only tests you can do, but they may help you discover that the techniques required are not beyond learning if you give them serious time and attention. The information here has been checked as thoroughly as possible, but new advances may make some data obsolete. This list is not intended to take the place of consultation with a physician. Instead, it is designed as a guide to help you monitor present conditions, to enable more people to undertake preventive health-care regimes, and to foster greater awareness of the tremendous contribution good health can make to your enjoyment of life.

In order to record and track the results of your own testing, consider starting a notebook. The best kind is a loose-leaf variety, so that pages may be lifted out and placed elsewhere in the book when the need to regroup data arises. When logging the information gathered from testing, the following should be carefully recorded *each time!*

—the date and time of the test, including the hour and the minute [Some tests should be done early in the morning, *before* having breakfast, others before moving around too much.]

—the name of the test

—the name of the person who worked with you on the testing

—a notation of what you had to eat before the test, specify the quantity
—the results of the test
—the estimated "normal" for that particular kind of test
[Remember to add the title, author and date of publication of the book you used to determine the "normal" you describe. This information will be helpful in case you decide to take your problem to a doctor later on. It will explain why you felt the results you arrived at were not "normal." It is important to realize that very few medical tests give 100 percent proof of the presence or absence of a disease. In addition, a considerable number of laboratory test results are erroneous. Never undergo potentially dangerous examinations, testing procedures, therapies or operations on the basis of a single test.]

Begin by checking your vital signs: temperature, blood pressure, pulse.

Temperature

Equipment: A thermometer can be purchased from any drug store or surgical supply house for about $3 to $5. Everyone should have one in the house, especially if there are children at home. There are two types: rectal and oral. Some good electronic thermometers are on the market, but they are fairly expensive.

Method: Directions for the proper use should be packaged with the thermometer when you buy it. Almost all of us have had our temperature taken, so the procedure is not a mystery.

Wash the thermometer in soap and cool water, and dry carefully. Grasp the thermometer by the high-reading end and shake it until the mercury column falls below the 95° F mark. Any reading will raise the mercury above that mark.

Place the thermometer under your tongue and keep it in your mouth for about three minutes, closing your lips around it carefully and making sure your teeth don't touch it. Remove the thermometer and take it to a strong light. Twist it until you can see where the mercury stopped. Turn it slightly and you will be able to read the numbers at that spot. The lower long-line reading indicates the degrees; the smaller lines indicate tenths of a degree.

Note: Don't use an oral thermometer for at least fifteen minutes after the patient has taken hot liquids.

A thermometer reading for children is usually taken rectally. The thermometer should remain in place for three minutes to permit the mercury to rise. If the temperature can not be taken rectally because of special conditions, you may have to have the child hold the thermometer tightly in the armpit.

This method is not always reliable and the thermometer should remain in the armpit at least five minutes to get as accurate a reading as possible.

Women determining the time of ovulation should take a temperature reading every morning upon waking, in order to detect the increase in temperature which occurs half-way between menstrual periods. This is the time of ovulation.

Results: There is not a definitive "normal" temperature reading, although 98.6° F or 37° C is usual. However, between 98° and 99.5° can be considered in the acceptable range. A fever is not necessarily an indication that something is wrong.

Some drugs cause a higher temperature, and increased activity also will raise the temperature.

A temperature taken rectally may be expected to be ½° to 1° higher than one taken orally, while one taken with the thermometer held in the armpit may be ½° to 1° lower. If the temperature is over 101° F, you should consult a physician.

When body temperature drops *below* normal, the condition is known as hypothermia. Often elderly people have lower than normal temperatures, especially if they live in cooler climates. Lower temperatures also may be related to circulatory problems or diabetes. Consistant hypothermia can be a sign of hypothyroidism. Hypothermia, when due to exposure to cold weather, can be very dangerous and should receive immediate care when noted.

Blood Pressure

There is little mystery in taking your blood pressure, so do not hesitate to learn how.

Equipment: You will need to buy or borrow a blood pressure measuring instrument. These range from electronic devices that give an instant digital readout of the results to the less expensive stethoscope and sphygmo-manometer. **Note:** Electronic devices sometimes give incorrect values. To check your unit have it compared to a mercury sphygmomanometer in your doctor's office. If it doesn't check out, send the unit back to be recalibrated by the factory that produced it.

A stethoscope will cost $15 or more. If you haven't used one before, buy the flat-surfaced diaphragm model rather than the bell-shaped one. The sphymomanometer, including the blood pressure "cuff" and the accompanying mercury gauge, will cost $25 or more. Two types of sphygmomanometers are available: the mercury-column type for home use and the aneroid model. The aneroid type is more convenient, more durable and less expensive. These instruments may be purchased at a surgical or hospital supply store. Many retail pharmacies carry them also. In the California-based magazine, *Medical Self-Care*, you will find ads for inexpensive implements. Their address is Post Office Box 717, Inverness, California 94937.

Instruction booklets are usually included with the instruments, but if they are not or the instructions are not clear enough, you should communicate with the manufacturer directly. Or you might choose to buy *How Your Blood Pressure is Measured*, published by W. A. Baum Co., Inc., of Copake, New York 11726. Other books on the subject are available as well.

Method: Rest comfortably for fifteen or twenty minutes before starting. Then, with your elbow and forearm resting comfortably on a flat surface, palm facing upward, wrap the cloth of the cuff around the upper part of your arm, snugly but not too tightly. Continue wrapping in the same direction and secure by tucking it in comfortably. Put the ends of the stethoscope into your ears gently, making sure that the ear pieces are curved forward so they go into the ears easily. Grasp the listening piece lightly and press it gently against the inside curve of the elbow. Close the valve that is just below the bulb for inflating the cuff, then pump air into the cuff, inflating it, but not too tightly. Keep the bell of the stethoscope pressed against the arm while you open the valve slowly. The air in the cuff will seep out. Then you will hear the sound of the heartbeat. The first sound is the systolic pressure reading. Allow the air to continue seeping out until the sound disappears; this point is the diastolic pressure reading.

The two sides of the heart beat alternately. The auricles beat first, then the ventricles. The part of the cardiac cycle during which the heart relaxes and the ventricles are filling is called the diastole. The period of contraction is called the systole. Thus, we all have two kinds of blood pressure—systolic and diastolic. Diastolic pressure is the lower of the two figures (as in 120/80). Here, 80 is the low pressure level in the arteries during the "runoff" period when the heart is relaxing. The figures record the number of millimeters the column of mercury is raised by the force of your blood pressure.

Results: No reading is normal for everyone, but between 100 and 140 is considered average for systolic pressure. Blood pressure rises with activity, such as standing up, and falls with rest. It also rises with anger, fright and other strong emotions. Sometimes blood pressure jumps rather sharply after menopause.

In familiar surroundings and under average conditions your reading will probably be closer to your usual norm. If the numbers seem to be high, check again. Get in touch with your doctor if the reading remains high.

Heart

Equipment: To check your heart rate, you will need the stethoscope you bought for checking your blood pressure, as well as a watch with a second hand.

Method: Using the stethoscope, you may count the rate of your heartbeat. Put the ear-pieces into your ears and adjust them until they are comfortable. Try listening to other things in the house first, like running water in a pipe, or a child's heartbeat. Then place the bell of the stethoscope about an inch and a half below the left nipple and in the space between two ribs. Count the beats for fifteen seconds and then multiply by four to get the number of beats per minute. Use a watch with a second hand to make sure the count is correctly measured. You can do a double check by counting for fifteen seconds and multiplying by four, and then check by counting for the entire minute.

Your pulse can also be taken without the stethoscope by pressing your index finger or middle finger on your wrist, just behind the hill of the thumb. Use the watch to monitor the time.

Results: If you have a fever, your pulse rate may be affected. Also, if you exercise strenuously just before the test, your rate may be faster.

The pulse rate for children is higher than for adults, and slower in a large person than in a small one. You might remember this way: The pulse rate is fast in a bird and very slow in an elephant. It will be higher if you are standing than sitting. Eating and drinking also will alter the pulse rate. Your pulse rate decreases when you are sleeping or resting, whether you have a fever or not; certain drugs also will alter the rate.

Seventy-two may be considered an average rate, but a normal adult can have a resting rate of 50 to over 90. An infant may have a rate of 130, and an 80-year old may have a rate of 60. A "normal" rate for an adult is usually in the 70s.

Circulation

The feet and hands feel cold when they are not getting sufficient blood. Fright can induce small spasms of the smaller arteries in the skin. If you develop cramps in the calf of one or both legs when walking fast, stopping for a few minutes may relieve them. Walking a great deal is encouraged if you experience problems of this sort with your legs; gently massaging the entire limb can help relieve the pain.

However, there is always the possibility of Buerger's disease in which the arteries and veins of the arms and legs are affected. The only treatment for the fatigue, pain in the feet, and sometimes ulceration or gangrene of Buerger's disease is absolute and complete abstinence from tobacco *in all forms*. Diagnosis of this illness, especially for smokers, is very important, since treatment is bed rest rather than the walking recommended for ordinary cramps.[1]

Mouth and Throat

The mouth is an area that can reveal significant health problems before they reach crisis proportions, if the proper signals are noted. The mouth and gums reveal when people are not getting an adequate diet. The tongue may show signs of anemia, and bleeding gums may signal infection, vitamin C deficiency or some blood diseases.

In the elderly, osteoporosis can extend to the bones of the mouth, resulting in loosening of the teeth. When the tonsils and soft palate of the mouth are affected and you experience a general feeling of lassitude and tiredness, examine these areas carefully. If there seems to be a growth of any kind, see your doctor promptly.

The mouth is also a good signpost to metal poisoning such as excessive mercury, aluminum, copper, lead or silver. The prognosis is good if the offending materials are identified and eliminated from your diet or environment.

Equipment: You will need a high-intensity pen-sized flashlight, a mirror and either a spoon with a smooth handle or a tongue depressor.

Method: The smooth handle of a spoon, warmed slightly under hot running water, will be more comfortable for you than a tongue depressor. Facing the mirror, open your mouth. Grasping the cup end of the spoon, turn it over and use the handle to push your tongue down. Position the flashlight so that you can examine your throat.

Results: When you have an infection, your throat will be red and may have patches of yellow or white in the rear portion. Gums which seem to be overgrown may signify that the patient has been taking medication for treatment of epilepsy for a long period of time. This should be carefully monitored.

The most common bacterial sore throat, familiarly called "strep throat" (for "streptococcus" throat) almost invariably is accompanied by fever. If you suspect you have strep throat, err on the side of caution and have a doctor take a culture. This is quickly and easily done by lightly pressing a sterile cotton swab into the infected area of the throat, stroking the cotton tip across the infection and then rubbing it on a Petri dish. This deposits the throat bacteria onto gelatin where it will grow. After the culture is obtained, the containers are turned over to a laboratory which will report the type of bacteria causing the problem. The doctor will then be able to prescribe an antibiotic to control the infection.

However, if this is another in a series of throat infections, the doctor may suggest you take the sample yourself and buy a Petri dish already prepared with agar gel. This can be purchased from a local pharmaceutical supply house. In that case, you should also buy sterile swabs. Stroke lightly across the infected area of your throat, then across the agar in the dish. Cover the culture immediately to prevent contamination from airborne bacteria and to assure that the throat culture is predominant. Then take the container to the doctor's office or laboratory, where they will identify the bacteria.

You run little risk in taking this kind of sample and experience little inconvenience.

Rashes in the mouth may be associated with measles and scarlet fever among other illnesses. Excessive saliva in the mouth may be the result of irritation from foods or drugs. Swelling of one of the glands that produce saliva could be cat-scratch disease. The prognosis for the disease is excellent, with minimal treatment.[2]

A canker sore is an open lesion of the lips or mouth, and can accompany a fever. A *chancre* is a much more serious problem. Chancre is associated with syphilis and usually appears on the penis or vagina, though it can also appear on the lip, tongue or within the mouth or throat, especially as the result of oral sex. The chancre itself is painless and hard with a soft center, and will disappear in one to four weeks whether or not the disease is treated. This is the primary stage, and if treatment is prompt and thorough at this time, an excellent prognosis is possible. However, if you have a mucous patch anywhere in the tissues of the mouth, also associated with a fever, sore throat and listlessness, the syphilis can be more serious but will have a good prognosis only if promptly treated. Give this immediate attention! Get to your doctor or hospital clinic right away.

Eyes

Equipment: The pen-light used to examine your throat will be helpful for examining the pupils of the eyes. This is the only piece of equipment you will need.

Method: Ask another person to lift the flashlight up and shine it into your face toward your eyes. The pupils should constrict when light is flashed on them. The whites should be bright and clear. If the areas that should be white are red or have tracings of red lines through the area, you may have an infection.

Next, measure the distance from your eyes to a book or newspaper as you read comfortably. This should be about twelve to eighteen inches. If it is more or less than that, you may need glasses or your glasses may need to be changed.

Another test is to have someone hold a finger perpendicular to the floor about three feet in front of your face, while you stand facing each other. Then, without moving your head, watch as your tester's finger moves to the right, and then to the left. Try this at distances of twelve and twenty-four inches. Your eyes should move easily, following the movement of the finger.

Close your eyes and touch your eyeballs through the eyelids. Very, very soft eyeballs may suggest Vitamin A deficiency or dehydration.

When foreign bodies get in your eye, be careful in removing the matter. If it is just dust, lift the upper lid over the lower one very carefully and roll the eye from side to side. This should do it.

If the trouble is sand or other particles, put your entire face into clean water and open your eyelids under the water, rolling your eyeballs.

Larger particles should be removed with great care, and would be handled best by the nearest pharmacist, physician's assistant or doctor. Large pieces of matter can scratch the eyeball badly, so immediate professional care is essential.

In the event of congestion of the eyelids, you may use a cold compress to relieve the condition. Wring out a cloth in ice-water or put the cloth on ice to chill it and then apply it over your closed eyes and cheeks.

If you have pus in your eyes, treat the matter *very* carefully, so that there is no chance for additional infection. It is best *not* to consider self-treatment for this condition. You can apply cold compresses when there is pain. Use hot compresses to help drain a sty on the eyelid and increase the supply of blood to the eye area. Once again, if there is pus, *do not try* to treat this yourself. Not only might you spread your own infection but you run the danger of infecting others in the same household who use the same tools or implements.

Eyestrain from overuse of the eyes may be relieved with a warm solution of an over-the-counter preparation such as *Hypotears* or *Visine*.

Many people complain of seeing little pieces of matter floating across their line of vision. This condition does not necessarily mean there is anything wrong with the eyes. Doctors call the sensation by its Latin name which translates "flying flies." The condition is caused by tissue particles floating in the fluid inside the eyeball. If the condition worsens, however, it could signify trouble inside the eye, and you should consult an ophthalmologist.

When someone has had a head injury, the pupils of the eyes are likely to be dilated (opened up) and will not respond to the presence of light. In this case, it is *urgent* that the individual be taken to the nearest hospital emergency room.

If one or both of your eyes wander, or eye-drift occurs (i.e., the eye seems to be all right one moment, then after being used intensely for a while, it seems to drift to one side), you have a muscle weakness. You may do exercises to strengthen these muscles. Most involve hand-eye coordination, such as stringing beads in a sequence. Additional exercises can be designed by a creative orthoptist.[3]

Eyes are one of the most sensitive parts of the body, and you should take great care to prevent even the mildest injury. The reaction of the pupils to light is most significant in evaluating injuries to certain areas of the brain. If the patient has been taking drugs, the pupils may not respond to light. Be sensitive to the drops you use, discard them immediately if they do not soothe. Cosmetics, creams and pollution may be irritating or drying to your eyes. People over forty should have their eyes checked regularly for glaucoma.

Ears

Checking your ears is a problem. It is impossible to check your own ears, and getting someone with the same enthusiasm for the job might be difficult. In addition, it may be difficult for an untrained person to interpret an ear exam. However, the testing can be done easily and cheaply, so don't fail to include it in your self-examination program.

Equipment: Speculums for examining the ears may be purchased at a pharmacy or a surgical supply store for $15 to $30. If you write for a catalog from *Medical Self-Care*, you will find they have them too. When ordering, make sure to specify that the speculum is for the ears. You will also need a high-intensity pen-sized flashlight.

Method: For a good view of the ear canal, grasp the earlobe with the thumb and middle finger and pull forward. Then bring the second finger forward against the middle of the ear. The canal is then straightened out sufficiently for a clear view.

Put the speculum into the canal and look for brown or black wax. Hearing difficulties may be caused by heavy wax. In fact, you may suspect wax as the problem when you find the television sound turned up too loud. If wax is present, put a couple of drops of 3 percent peroxide in the ear canal. It will soften and bubble out the wax. If wax is heavy, do a little at a time for three or four days. Do not try to remove wax with a cotton swab, as injury may result.

If there is no wax present, the ear drum will look shiny and pearly white or light pink. This is normal. If it is infected, it will be partly red. If the color is bluish, it may mean there is fluid in the middle ear.

If inserting the speculum causes pain, stop the examination immediately. This might be a sign of difficulty with the ear or the ear canal, which is very curved and difficult to examine.[4] Contact your doctor for an examination as soon as you can! Infections of the external ear canal should be referred to your doctor as well.

If you experience dizziness or fainting after an ear injury, you may have difficulty with the part of the ear responsible for balance. To check this out, stand with your feet together and close your eyes. If you have a sensation of "vertigo"—defined as dizziness or a sensation of moving around in space—you may have a problem with the middle ear. This too needs the care of a doctor, and the sooner it is attended to, the better the chances of getting it under control quickly, cheaply and completely.

Urine Check

As many as twenty tests can be done with a single urine sample. Although I will not discuss all of them at this time, these tests will be discussed further in the following chapters.

The first specimen in the morning is the most useful for testing, and it should be a midstream specimen. That means that you begin urination, stop midway, and then collect the specimen. The urine should be tested as soon as conveniently possible, but no later than fifteen minutes to half an hour after it is produced. Try to expose the specimen to as little light as possible.

Equipment: You will need a wide-mouth jar to catch the urine and one of several kinds of paper testing strips (dipsticks) such as Chemstrip 9 or N-Multistix SG. These may be purchased in most pharmacies for about $4 to $6. Determine ahead of time that the particular tests you want done are possible with the product you purchase.

Method: Sterilize a wide-mouth container or jar by boiling it in water that covers it completely for about twenty minutes. Remove the jar from the boiling water with tongs if possible, making sure you don't touch the inside. Allow it to air dry.

A woman should spread the lips of her vagina and wash the whole area carefully with warm water and soap, then rinse. Don't dry. Holding the lips of the vagina apart, urinate into the jar. An uncircumcised man should pull back the foreskin and wash the head of the penis with warm soap and water, then rinse, and urinate into the jar.

Results: The dipsticks are produced to detect certain substances in the urine and to indicate, among other conditions, infection, drug abuse, the activity of hormones, proteins, sugar and how the body uses acetone and other chemicals. Acetone is formed when the body breaks down fats, and occurs in severe diabetes. It is also associated with high fevers, starvation and aspirin drug use. The papers that come with the dipsticks explain how they may be used, with warnings that results which deviate from acceptable standards should be referred to a physician promptly. Certain foods, drugs and conditions such as burns and shocks can affect the readings.

Dipsticks should be handled carefully and kept in a dry, cool place for storage once they have been opened or they will no longer be reliable.

Consult *Do-It-Yourself Medical Testing*, by Cathey Pinckney and Edward R. Pinckney, for more complete information about urine testing.

Feces Test

Equipment: The American Cancer Society runs a campaign to distribute folders to be used to take samples of feces over a two-day period to check for blood in the stool. You may contact your local American Cancer Society chapter to request a brochure. There is sometimes a modest charge for the folders. The society will give you the address to which you should send the samples for analysis. Kits for doing this test at home are also available in local pharmacies for about $8.

To get a correct test reading, you should avoid eating fish or meat for at least three days prior to the test. If you don't observe this caution, you may get an incorrect positive result.

Method: Directions for use of the kit are simple and accompany the package. Toothpicks and treated tissues are usually included with the packet. On two consecutive days, a tiny sample of feces should be taken by using one of the toothpicks or swabs and placing it on a small piece of tissue in the folder. After the second sample is taken in the same manner, the folder is slipped into the accompanying envelope and sent off for checking.
Results: Results will be sent directly to you if you include a self-addressed stamped envelope or a self-addressed post card.

Breast Self-Examination

A good deal of publicity has attended the campaign to urge women to examine their breasts regularly. Unfortunately the publicity has been aimed solely at women, and only women are pictured in the illustrative examples. Nevertheless, both *men and women* should do this testing regularly.

The consistency of the breasts changes during the menstrual cycle, so examinations should be done about the same time each month, a few days to a week after your period. You will become familiar with the shape and texture of your body, and may detect anything unusual more quickly than a doctor would.

Equipment: Little equipment is required for self-examination of the breasts: only a mirror for the first part of the examination, and a bed for the second part.
Method: First, stand in front of your mirror with your hands at your side. Raise your hands over your head, then move them to a position firmly cupping your hips. Note any differences between your breasts' shape, such as a flattening or a bulge in one but not in the other, a sore on or near the nipple, an inverted nipple or puckered skin.

Then, lie on your back on the bed. Raise one arm over your head and, using the flat of the fingers on the opposite hand, trace small circles until the entire breast has been covered. The most common location of tumors is between the nipple and the armpit, so it is necessary to give a little more attention to that area.[5]

Charts are offered free of charge by the American Cancer Society with specific directions on how to do breast examinations and how often. They describe the circular motions to be followed and the lying-down position that will help to highlight a lump if one is present. Most cities and towns in the United States have a chapter of the American Cancer Society, but if you prefer to write for your copy of the booklet, the address is 777 Third Avenue, New York, New York 10017.

Results: Lumps in the breast are not always malignant. In fact, most lumps in the breast are *not* cancerous. Remember that anyone sensitive to caffeine, who eats chocolate regularly, drinks large quantities of soft drinks, coffee, tea or cocoa may develop a non-malignant lump in the breast. If you discover a lump, visit your doctor. *If lengthy treatment or surgery is suggested by your doctor, don't fail to consult at least one other physician.* Incorrect diagnosis is not uncommon. When biopsies are frozen and examined hastily, while the patient is still under anesthesia, the error rate is very high. There is rarely a good reason for immediate surgery and you should be offered the opportunity to decide what type of treatment you would prefer to undergo, if any.

Pregnancy Test

Equipment: Many pregnancy tests are available at the local pharmacy without a doctor's prescription. The cost is $10 to $20.

Method: Sterilize a wide-mouth container or jar by boiling it in water that covers it completely for about twenty minutes. Remove the jar with tongs if possible, making sure not to touch the inside. Allow it to air dry.

Spread the lips of the vagina and wash the whole area with warm water and soap, then rinse. Don't dry. Holding the lips of the vagina apart, urinate into the jar.

Results: The test will react to the presence of the hormone that increases when a woman is pregnant, and sediment will accumulate at the bottom of the jar.

The test itself comes with explicit instructions. It may not, however, warn that some foods, liquids, medicines or drugs can affect the results. It might be a good idea to have a period of fasting before using the test kit.[6]

The tests are only 80 to 95 percent accurate, so bear in mind that 5 to 20 percent of the time the results may be negative when they should be positive, or positive when they should be negative. Remember, too, that the hormone level may not be high enough yet to register.

You should confirm your results by having a doctor perform the same test.

Alcoholism

Alcoholism is a potentially fatal disease which can cause deterioration in body organs as well as in brain function. Every effort should be made to interrupt the drinking pattern cycle of an alcoholic at the earliest stage possible.

Medication is available that will make drinking a trauma situation—if the alcoholism is caught early enough. The patient must be thoroughly examined by a physician before this pill is prescribed, since it can severely strain the body if deterioration has begun.

Equipment: The Johns Hopkins University Hospital Alcoholism Screening Test or the Self-Administered Alcoholism Screening Test should be used to determine the likelihood of being alcoholic. Testing by questionnaire is considered fairly accurate for finding future alcoholics.[7] The Johns Hopkins Test is described by Pinckney and Pinckney in *Do-It-Yourself Medical Testing*, and the second test—or one similar to it—is available through your local Alcoholics Anonymous group. Their number is in your telephone book. Other tests are available through local drug-help clinics and associations which are often located in easily-accessible areas. The tests consist of twenty-five to thirty-five questions.

Drunkenness: There are several ways of testing for drunkenness. The breathalyzer is used to analyze air breathed into it. Urine testing can also be done. With the urine test, you must first urinate and empty your bladder, then wait about twenty to thirty minutes before giving the sample to be tested. The sample will then reflect the true quantity of alcohol in the system.

Legal intoxication levels differ from state to state. Alcoholic beverages come in many different proofs, which must be considered when using the term liquor. Vodka distilled in the United States, for instance, has a very high proof, over 190. Mescal and four-year-old tequila are marketed at 86 to 100 proof. Also, proof can be as low as 50 for some of the more exotic liqueurs. Creme de Cacao, for example, is 50 to 54 proof, while Golden Irish Mist is 80 proof. Beer generally is under 14 proof and wine varies between 20 and 28. Ten ounces of high proof liquor showing 0.4 percent of alcohol in the blood can produce stupor or coma, and twelve ounces taken at one time can produce serious consequences, even death.[8]

Aside from the problem of testing for whether a person is too drunk to drive properly, it is important to determine the degree of intoxication if a person is unconscious or in a coma because of an accident. Under these conditions, a blood test will often be done, which will test the enzymes or the folic acid.[9] This type of testing is also used to differentiate between an overdose of tranquilizers or antihistamines. There are also instances in which environmental toxicity can produce symptoms in delicate or sensitive individuals that appear to be alcohol related.

Hair Mineral Analysis

Do not overlook the possibility of having your hair sample analyzed. Hair analysis will test for calcium, chromium, zinc, aluminum, lead, mercury and other chemicals. The analysis may even establish whether the relationships between the types of minerals in your body are satisfactory. Exposure to toxic metals that occurred months earlier may be reflected through hair analysis, whereas blood and urine testing usually show only those minerals present at the time of testing. This method is frequently used to determine lead poisoning in children. Although tests can be performed on hair from anywhere on the body, most laboratories prefer a sample cut off close to the scalp at the nape of the neck. It is sometimes recommended that pubic hair be used to minimize the possibility of exterior contamination.

New self-testing items are constantly being introduced which may make diagnosis and treatment simpler, safer and cheaper. It is worth the time and trouble to keep abreast of these new developments. For instance, a new device for detecting breast cancer in women is available. This "detector" consists of two plastic discs containing heat-sensitive plastic chemicals that are to be worn inside the bra for about fifteen minutes per month. A color change indicates an abnormality, necessitating the proper follow-up testing.

The device may be costly, however, a club or a women's center might purchase one and make it available for a nominal fee to many women. Used in this manner, it will cost less than the present types of breast screening and hopefully will reduce the number of women who need exploratory surgery, or who lose entire breasts, adjacent nerves, lymph glands and muscles.[10]

The detector's false-negative rate (the number of times the test indicates "no" when it should say "yes") is about 13 percent; the false-positive rate (the times the test shows a "yes" when it should be "no") is about the same. The results of the testings have been compared to the thermographic breast test findings that are being done to replace harmful x-rays. Of the people diagnosed as being "suspicious" as a result of the thermographic testing, about a third have developed cancer within five years. These women were considered to be in the "high risk" group.[11]

For the first time, women may have a chance to get an early and accurate diagnosis using safe, non-invasive techniques.

Most women are still sent to a laboratory for x-ray testing. Most people are unaware of the possibility of having a thermograph instead of an x-ray. Widespread use of the traditional x-ray equipment has probably prevented the new diagnostic machine from becoming widely known. The thermograph is an instrument that records the heated places in the body and produces an immediate picture. It was developed as a result of the observation that when a part of the body has been injured and is trying to heal itself, that area is considerably warmer than its surrounding tissue. Originally the thermograph was designed to verify back and neck injuries, but it soon became useful in locating "hot spots" in other areas of the body, particularly the breasts. Thermograms do not diagnose breast cancer, but they do indicate *probabilities*.

Doctors who claim that low voltage mammograms are the best method of picking up small very early cancers of the breasts, and that x-rays do better than the thermograph does, however, agree that 90 percent of breast tumors are really found during regular patient self-examination, and not by mammograms or x-rays. Those women with a family or medical history that indicates routine examinations are advisable, should be reassured that newer mammography machines deliver very low radiation and are becoming available nationwide.

In assessing your condition or the condition of others, don't fail to investigate the possibility that the "mental symptoms" a person is showing might be evidence of a very real physical disorder. The fact that the person has become hostile, quick-tempered, withdrawn or indifferent, for instance, could indicate diabetes, thyroid condition or heart disease. If there has been a severe personality change, if the person is becoming harder to get along with, suggest extensive and conclusive testing before coming to the conclusion that there is something mentally wrong.

Cathey Pinckney and Edward R. Pinckney, M.D. have recently published two comprehensive books about medical tests. *Do-It-Yourself Medical Testing* and *The Patient's Guide to Medical Tests* suggest "normal values" for test results. All the tests a doctor might order are explained in very readable form. *Do-It-Yourself Medical Testing* will help you evaluate the results of your own testing as well.

In addition to your own testing, you may take advantage of tests offered either free of charge or for a nominal sum by the American Red Cross. These tests are usually for anemia, height and weight, visual acuity, glaucoma, hearing, heart disease and diabetes. There is a charge for optional blood testing which gives readings on cholesterol, liver and kidney function, gout and triglycerides. For information on tests available in your area, contact your local Red Cross chapter. If they have not had a drive of this type recently, perhaps you can volunteer to help arrange one.

None of the tests you have taken yourself, however, should take the place of checking in with your physician, so that you may work together to attack the problems you have found. When your results seem to be out of line or are hard to interpret, do the test again. Record the information for the second test—and the third, if necessary—below or on the next page of your notebook so that the results may be compared easily.

In many cases, the test your doctor will do is identical, or fairly similar to what you have already done for yourself. The results should not vary greatly. If there is a great difference between the results of the doctor's test and your results, consider that:

—You may have done the test incorrectly.

—You may have read the results incorrectly.

—The person who evaluated the results of the test in your doctor's office might not be your doctor, but an employee who may not be as qualified to do so. Check on this; it is important and more prevalent than you may realize.

—The "normal" you are using may differ from the standard the doctor is using. Exchange sources with your doctor and decide which source is more recent and accurate.

—It is possible the equipment the doctor has been using is worn out and obsolete.

Remember, very few medical tests give 100 percent proof of the presence or absence of a disease, and the results are subject to a number of errors caused by the machine and/or the operator.

Never depend upon a single test result if you still do not feel well. Have the test done a second and even a third time, by another laboratory, by another doctor, or by yourself. *Never undergo potentially dangerous examinations, testing procedures or therapies on the basis of a single test.*[12]

When government sources tested laboratories for accuracy, they found that one out of every seven tests was invalid[13]; either the results were incorrect or the wrong tests were ordered for the suspected disorder. If your blood, urine and feces were taken for testing at the laboratory, consider the fact that up to fifteen tests could be done with the materials taken. In this there is a possibility of having at least one or two incorrect results. There have been reports of electrocardiogram machines being incorrectly calibrated, of thousands of sphygmomanometers giving wrong readings, and of x-ray machines being run by unqualified and inexperienced people.

Be comforted. Your test results are likely to be as accurate as the doctor's; the book you used, (copyrighted or revised within the last few years), is likely to be as up-to-date as the book used by your doctor. In fact, your tests are likely to be more scrupulously performed. The results, also carefully noted, are more likely to produce readings that cannot be challenged for accuracy. Even the American Medical Association confirms that the tests you do for yourself are often as accurate at locating or detecting curable diseases as the ones given at the doctor's office. However, only the doctor can write the prescription or order the surgery that your condition might require.

For many years we have been told to have a yearly examination to stay healthy, but recently some medical people have been saying that our health conditions today are far worse, rather than better.[14]

The false hope that something can be done about any illness caught early enough has dropped a pall of guilt over parents whose children are monitored with apprehension, and over spouses who watch their mates ail and sometimes die. There is no way to make up for bad eating habits, excessive drinking, smoking or jobs with tremendous amounts of stress and toxic exposure, e.g., asbestos, radiation, insecticides, dusts, silica.

If the results of your own tests alert you to the possibility of problems, plan to visit your family physician. The re-emerging field of family medicine can bring a rounded and holistic presence to the problem of diagnosis.

Perhaps with enough impetus from you and me, patient-education materials will become more available and the enormous amounts of money spent on treatment and diagnosis will be balanced with more effective education for healthful living and care of an individual's own health.

NOTES

1. James Dunlap, *Medical Negligence: The Uncontrolled Killer*, p. 14.
2. S.N. Bhaskar, *Synopsis of Oral Pathology*, p. 69.
3. Robison, D. Harley, *Pediatric Ophthalmology*, 2nd ed., p. 1302.
4. Keith Sehnert and Howard Eisenberg, *How to Be Your Own Doctor— Sometimes*, pp. G122–123.
5. Boston Women's Health Collective, *Our Bodies, Ourselves*, p. 127.
6. Cathey Pinckney and Edward R. Pinckney, *Do-It-Yourself Medical Testing*, pp. 20, 21.
7. Pinckney and Pinckney, *The Patient's Guide to Medical Tests*, p. 117.
8. Ibid., p. 7.
9. Ibid., p. 8.
10. Robison D. Harley, *Pediatric Ophthalmology*, p. 3049.
11. Ibid., p. 3048.
12. Pinckney and Pinckney, *Patient's Guide*, p. xi.
13. Ibid., p. xii.
14. Michael L. Culbert, *Save Your Life*, p. 67.

2

Finding and Assessing Your Doctor

If the results of some of the tests you have done are troubling you, only a confirmation of the findings—or an explanation—will settle your fears. The next step is to see a doctor.

You are torn between visiting the doctor who has been the mainstay for the family and revealing the tests you did at home, and forgetting the whole thing. Don't hesitate to change doctors. The change might make all the difference in the world. The physician who has cared for you a good part of your life and could be a good "friend," could overlook symptoms with serious consequences. A cursory examination is worse than none at all. It gives a false sense of having done what was necessary and of having considered all options.[1] To further complicate making the decision, women sometimes feel that doctors think they exaggerate their illnesses, or that they visit the doctor to get attention. The fact is, the medical profession in the United States is overwhelmingly male, with women making up 11.6 percent of the profession.[2]

In assessing your doctor, consider the following questions: Is your doctor really sincere about determining what is wrong with you? Have you been given a vague explanation or a recommendation for a "tonic" rather than a thorough examination? Have your questions been put off with an invitation to "let me do the worrying"?

All of these are difficult assessments to make, but they are important. Your doctor is the only person who can confirm a diagnosis you may have reached by yourself, or to suggest one if you have not. Only your physician may suggest and prescribe medication, discuss the possibility of surgery or reassure you officially that nothing is wrong.

So, square your shoulders and take the plunge. It is time to find, choose and evaluate a doctor. But before you go to a doctor, there are things you should decide to do to help determine the direction of the examination. You should determine the questions you will want answered, consider the possibility of alternate diagnoses, and demand an explanation of any medications prescribed and any terms you don't understand. You are paying for all of this; why not demand the best possible service? You can in the grocery store. You can in the clothing store. Why not in the doctor's office?

Then how do you choose a doctor? There are several ways to go.

If you are going to a new community, perhaps the doctor you were fond of and with whom you had a good rapport could recommend a physician in the area. Don't hesitate to get in touch with your previous doctor by mail or telephone to ask for a recommendation. It is likely that your records will be sent promptly to the person recommended. Then your new doctor will have an idea of your previous medical care.

The American Academy of Family Physicians can help you find a family practice physician. They can provide a free list of family physicians in your area. Their address is American Academy of Family Physicians, 1740 West Second Street, Kansas City, Missouri 64114.

Another source is your neighbors. They will be glad to share this information with you, although their advice must be weighed carefully. People have different priorities when judging doctors. Some people are most concerned with a doctor's manner; others care only about the issue of competence.

You might telephone the local Medical Society for a recommendation, although this resource is limited. They will merely disclose where you can find the nearest professional directories which will list the physicians in your area in alphabetical order, the schools they attended, the places they practiced, their ages, addresses, and telephone numbers. After you have scanned the list, you may then choose to call a younger doctor, more recently graduated and only lately established in practice. This person might not have a great deal of experience, but is likely to know the newer discoveries, and be more attentive to your needs, so as to build up a practice. On the other hand, you could choose an older, more established physician, with a wider practice and more years of experience. The *Directory of Medical Specialists* contains thousands of listings of medical specialists in each state, county, and city across the nation. The directory will include how long the doctor has been practicing, and how long s/he has specialized in the chosen field. You may make your choice with relation to how far from home or work you would want to travel for an office visit.

The Medical Society will not make any kind of recommendation, however. They will not help you select one doctor over any others and will not discuss competence, fees, or adequacy of training.

If you have the opportunity to do so, you might ask members of the medical profession who they go to. You could ask a doctor, a nurse or a social worker. In some instances, personal bias may lead a medical professional to recommend a physician who is insensitive to your needs. Some doctors are not receptive to patients who require explanations, ask for alternative diagnoses, intimate that they are not drug takers and believe in the usefulness of alternative therapies.

There is no clearing house for information that can alert you to the dangers of dealing with insensitive or even incompetent physicians. Doctors who have committed excesses have been, and continue to be, free to move from state to state to practice their profession.[3] Each state has its own licensing procedures, so that negligence charges in one state can be erased forever by moving to an adjacent one! In California, a judge can—and often does—order that information incriminating a doctor be kept from the licensing authorities of the state.[4]

One state has only two investigators to police its nineteen thousand doctors. Compare the two investigators they have in the medical sphere with the seven for real estate complaints and the four who investigate cosmetological procedures. Which would involve a more life-threatening situation, investigating doctors or real estate operations?[5]

Stories of medical incompetence surface from time to time. It is not clear that the medical profession has begun to clean its own house by acting against its members who have acted irresponsibly and are still practicing medicine. To this end, try to find people who have been patients of the doctor you have decided to see.

In general, those of us who have found doctors practicing in groups have had more satisfying patient-doctor relationships. Groups of physicians seem to present to each other increased tolerance for challenge. Doctors practicing independently may miss this stimulus. With an independent practitioner you might miss out on having a doctor on call when your own doctor is ill, on vacation or unavailable at the time of your emergency. All group practice setups do not necessarily require that a patient take whichever doctor is available at the time of the visit. You may, with many group practices, choose the doctor who will be your constant consultant—except during the emergencies when s/he is not available.

It is generally felt that a poor doctor will not stay in a group of this kind, since the constant consultation requires that each doctor make a fair contribution to the knowledge and cooperation of the entire group. The cooperative funding that group practice doctors provides for their physical surroundings often extends to providing sufficient nursing and para-professional help, as well as providing expensive equipment. In addition, patient-education facilities are likely to be better. The American Group Practice Association, as well as other companies, provides written, taped and videotaped information for the instruction of their patients.[6]

Another alternative is the Health Maintenance Organization (HMO). The government has been encouraging development of these organizations. These are prepaid medical care groups with many specialty physicians forming the nucleus of the organization. Not everyone has the option of belonging to an HMO, since many cities or towns have not yet established one. However, HMOs are moving into new areas all the time in an effort to help contain health costs and promote preventive medical programs. Some unfavorable publicity which has arisen about HMOs bears further investigation before taking it for the truth.

The largest of the HMOs have won themselves enviable reputations for speedy care, accurate diagnoses, and most important, fewer operations. The best known HMOs are The Harvard Community Health Plan (HCHP) in Boston, the Health Insurance Plan (HIP) in New York City and the Kaiser Permanente Plan in Los Angeles.

Choose the names of a few doctors you would consider using and then do not hesitate to telephone each office. Ask the secretary or nurse to answer some questions for you: Will the doctor take Medicare/Medicaid patients? Will s/he wait for the check to come from the government, or will s/he require a check from the patient at the end of the session? Ask if there is a schedule of fees for office visits, for certain types of procedures, for testing and surgery, and if itemized bills are provided.

These are some of the questions the People's Medical Society has been asking doctors as they form chapters and send out mailings to the health professionals in their areas. In a survey in Prince George's County, Maryland, made by the Health Research Group (a Nader Study Group) only 115 physicians out of 560 in the area responded to questions like these when they were telephoned.[7]

Don't forget that the attitude of the people in the front office or answering the telephone reflects the attitude of the doctor to a great degree. If you are annoyed or offended by their attitude, you may not be happy with their boss.

The nurse will usually prevent you from talking on the telephone directly with the doctor, even if you say it is an emergency. The nurse may advise you on taking medication if you call to say it is making you ill—sometimes with and sometimes without consulting the doctor—but trained to do so with the knowledge and consent of the doctor.

Think of it this way: you are paying your doctor from $25 to $50 per visit. How long does the doctor spend in the room with you? Ten minutes? Fifteen? More? Based on these fees for an average of fifteen minutes with you, his/her potential earnings will be around $100 to $200 per hour, or $600 to $1,200 per day—for a six-hour day. This does not include the sums billed Medicare or Medicaid for visits to patients already in the hospital, with whom little time may be spent.

If you are buying the time of someone who is in the quarter-million-dollar-a-year class, are you sure you aren't out of your milieu? If the answer is "no," then how much time do you think the doctor ought to give you . . .or wouldn't it be better to find some other physician who could give you less superficial care? If your doctor is seeing six to eight patients an hour, find another doctor. That is what is known in the profession as "cash register medicine."[8] Unless it is an emergency and the doctor must rush to the bedside of a patient already in the hospital, don't make it a practice to wait more than fifteen or twenty minutes for your care.

In negotiations for medical faculty salaries at a prominent teaching hospital, one negotiator contended that the doctors wanted a guaranteed yearly income of $700,000 to devote their time completely and exclusively to teaching in the medical school. However, the union representing the doctors insisted that they would settle for $220,000.[9]

It is difficult to discern whether prospective doctors keep up with the recent findings in their fields. At the time I was a medical librarian and in search of a grant from the National Library of Medicine for expansion of my library's collection, I sent out, with the approval of the hospital administration, about two hundred letters to doctors, social workers, nurses and social service organizations inviting them to make use of our services. Serving the neighborhood as well as our own staff would have enlarged the scope and coverage of our medical data considerably and would certainly have won for us the large grant we requested. None of the professionals were interested in hearing from our medical library on a regular basis about the new advances in their fields, from journals they might not have access to. Many states, responding to the appalling lack of attention to the newest advances in medicine by doctors, have required evidence of a certain amount of study from all physicians renewing their medical licenses.

Patients are usually at a great disadvantage when trying to evaluate a doctor or a particular kind of therapy, since few of us are informed about the appropriateness of the medical care we are receiving. In 1979, during a doctors' strike in Los Angeles, the mortality rate for the area dropped 20 percent. One doctor dryly commented that the death rate might have been even lower had surgeons in the county university hospitals participated in the strike.[10]

Some doctors will make an appointment for a ten- or fifteen-minute "get-acquainted" session, for which they charge the usual office fee. However, this is a worthwhile investment of time and money, and will prevent your going through a long physical examination with a doctor you realize you will not want to see again.[11]

The doctor's manner should put you at ease. If you are the kind of person who does not care whether you know how to spell the name of your illness or what it means, or if you are not concerned with the possible side-effects of the medication ordered for you, you may like an authoritative individual.

However, if you are the kind of person who wants to know a good many of the answers, do not stay with a doctor who resents a lot of questions or a request for an alternate diagnosis. Find one who is warm, willing to explain and makes an effort to relate to his/her patients.

During your brief visit, sit back and examine your doctor as seriously as you expect him/her to examine you. Does s/he seem sound of body and mind? Does s/he seem well-organized? Is the office clean and neat? Do you feel comfortable with this doctor? These issues may be an indication of the quality of care this doctor might provide. Incidentally, there are doctors who the American Medical Association suggests should not be practicing medicine.[12] Therefore, careful screening of your doctor is certainly justified.

Be prepared, if necessary, to write a check to cover the cost of the visit. The poorer you are, the less likely you will find a doctor willing to give you sufficient attention and care. It is becoming exceedingly rare for doctors to wait for their money until Medicare and/or Medicaid has cleared the claim.

If the doctor will visit with you for a few minutes first, before you go into a more comprehensive medical session, you will have a clearer idea of whether you can relate well to each other. Then, if you like what you have learned in your first contact, make the appointment that might be the beginning of a rewarding relationship.

Now that you are about to start with a new doctor, you should get your medical records from your previous physician. It will be instructive for you to look at your file, as well as helpful for your new doctor to see what kind of care you have needed in the past.[13]

NOTES

1. Isadore Rosenfeld, *The Complete Medical Exam*, p. 31.
2. *Statistical Abstract of the United States*, 1982-1983, 103rd edition. U.S. Department of Commerce, Bureau of the Census, Washington, D.C., 1982, pp. 912–913.
3. "License to Kill," *People's Weekly*, 26 July 1982, vol. 8, pp. 24–25.
4. James Dunlap, *Medical Negligence: The Uncontrolled Killer*, p. 20.
5. John H. Knowles, *Doing Better and Feeling Worse: Health in the United States*, p. 31.
6. Keith Sehnert, *How to Be Your Own Doctor—Sometimes.* p. 89.
7. Ibid., p. 89.
8. Ibid., p. 99.
9. "Union is Assailed on Medical Faculty Incomers," *New York Times*, Sunday, 29 August 1982, p. 48.
10. Sehnert, p. 101.
11. "License to Kill," *People's Weekly*, p. 24.
12. Dunlap, p. 84.
13. "Physician Opens Medical Records to His Patients," *Sarasota Herald Tribune*, 3 April 1985, p. XDS.

3

Visiting Your Doctor:
A Thorough Physical Exam

Two kinds of visits are described in this chapter. The first, hopefully, will last fifteen or twenty minutes at the most, and will familiarize you with the person for whom you are going to undress completely, subject yourself to intimate examination, and answer very personal questions. The other type of visit is the actual "thorough physical examination."

GETTING ACQUAINTED SESSION

During the "get-acquainted" session you will have an opportunity to talk in general terms about some of the things that will help make future visits more comfortable. You might also ask some questions, such as: May I bring a friend or relative into the examining room? Will you accept telephone calls occasionally, or will it be necessary for me to make an appointment to talk to you for a few minutes? Do you feel diet is intimately connected to good health? Will you prescribe generic drugs?

None of these queries are intended to embarrass, upset or challenge your doctor, but to give you, the patient, an idea of how willing and flexible the doctor is to meeting your needs. The graciousness and interest that the doctor shows in answering your questions should help you decide whether or not this is the physician you want to have on a continuing basis. Don't take on a doctor just because s/he has been recommended by someone else. If you have any inner misgivings, bow out gracefully and go on looking for "your" doctor.

If the short preliminary meeting you requested passed satisfactorily, you may make an appointment for the "thorough physical examination."

Preparations

List of Symptoms: In your notebook list the symptoms you have that made you want to see the doctor. This should be done over a period of a couple of days, so that information may be added as you think of it. Make a copy of your list to leave with the doctor to be kept as part of your file.

Note whether you have the symptoms at any particular time of the day, such as just after eating or just before bedtime.

Does anyone else in the family have this particular problem? In other words, is it possible that this condition runs in the family?

Did you eat anything strange lately? Did you eat a kind of food unfamiliar to you? Did you travel somewhere you have never been before? Did you recently wear clothing made of a fabric new to you, that might trigger an allergic reaction?

Were you taking any kind of medication when the symptoms began? Have you stopped taking it? Have the symptoms disappeared? Were you taking vitamins, tranquilizers, food supplements? If the answer is yes, mention which, how much and how often.

Is it possible that these new complaints are related to an earlier condition that was diagnosed and treated some time ago, or that was *not* diagnosed and treated but simply went away?

List of Medications: Make a list of medications you are currently taking on a regular basis. Put a check mark or star next to any medication this doctor prescribed for you in the past. Add to this section what condition or conditions were diagnosed at the time these medications were prescribed. Make any comments you wish next to the name or description of these medications: did the drug help the condition it was prescribed for, did it do nothing at all, did it hinder recovery?

Note whether too much medication was prescribed, which you probably had to throw away. This is unwarranted waste for you, but profit for the pharmaceutical company and for the drug store. If you mention it specifically it might not happen again.

In many states the name of the medication must appear on the bottle or jar. If it does not, just list the number, the date, the name of the doctor who prescribed it, and the address of the pharmacy. Bring the bottle with you when you go to the doctor's office; the medication can be identified for you if there is still one pill left in the jar. If there isn't, the doctor can call the drug store and ask them to look up their records.

Preparation for Tests: If the doctor is going to do a Pap smear, a woman should not douche; for a proctoscopy, you will need to have an enema about two hours before the examination. Find out whether you can have breakfast before you come or whether you should fast for twelve or twenty-four hours before the testing.

If you don't make this kind of preparation, the results of the tests might be skewed and a second visit would be necessary to complete the examination. You should call and ask the office if any preparations are necessary.

THOROUGH PHYSICAL EXAMINATION

After a short wait, you have gained the quiet and solemnity of the inner sanctum. There you are told to take off all your clothes. The small gown you are given has an opening at the back, and is barely big enough to wrap around you. Feeling at a tremendous disadvantage and undignified, you are now ready for that "thorough physical examination."

The doctor usually begins by compiling as complete a medical history as possible. You will be asked for information about your past illnesses and operations, the illnesses of your family members, the amount of alcoholic beverages you consume, whether or not you smoke, or if there are products in the environment at work or at home that could be affecting your health. You may even be asked which foods seem to make you ill or seem hard for you to digest. The doctor may inquire about your urinary and bowel movements. If you are a woman, your doctor will want a fairly complete gynecological history as well.

You will be questioned about your life in general, including a run-down of your daily habits. How well you sleep could be a clue to nervous tension, and your attitude toward life could indicate how well you might follow a prescribed regimen. This information will affect your prognosis (the doctor's evaluation of the chances for your recovery). Be calm and cooperative. A hurried or incomplete examination can sometimes lead to a misdiagnosis.[1] Refer to your notes in giving the doctor all the data you collected, because the possibility of error in diagnosis is tremendous and any help you can give is important. If you have not already done so, mention any drugs you are taking, as well as food supplements, vitamins or laxatives. Some of these are drugs too, and may make a difference in the assessment of your condition.

If you have been to this doctor before, or if you have brought your file from your previous physician, allow the doctor an opportunity to review your file while you wait patiently. A few doctors do not bother with this review, but it is important that your doctor does or you might find yourself taking medication upon medication intended to do opposite things, taking medication you are allergic to, or even taking double doses of the identical medication prescribed the last time.

Before leaving this portion of the examination, the doctor should review with you all the data you brought from home, symptom by symptom. The doctor will then have the opportunity to try to supplement the information by asking more questions: does leaning over, walking fast, or reaching for something overhead bring on the symptoms? Have you noticed changes in the symptoms over a period of time? Have they gotten worse? Better?

If you are a woman, however, mention that you are concerned, since identical symptoms have been known to be diagnosed differently for each sex. Doctors sometimes ascribe "empty nest syndrome" to the complaints of older women, then order tranquilizers. The weight gain that might signal alcoholism or kidney or heart failure in a man is sometimes written off as "mid-life crisis" in a woman.

After the history has been taken, the doctor will begin the "hands-on" portion of the exam. This is the point at which you might want to disclose your own test results.

Height and Weight: Your height and weight will be taken. There is no "ideal" weight for a particular height, because it is dependent upon the type of body build and the heaviness of inherited bone structure.

Temperature: Although the best and most accurate manner of taking temperature readings is rectally, it is rare that this is done with adults. The danger of children breaking the thermometer in their mouths makes it more prudent to take their temperature rectally. The "ideal" temperature is thought to be 98.6° F, although this too will vary.

Blood Pressure: With the publicity given hypertension (high blood pressure) recently, many people have become anxious about their blood pressure. This anxiety surfaces in the doctor's office when the cuff is placed on your arm and often causes the reading to be "high." Blood pressure readings can also vary when you are sitting down or standing up. If the readings are very high, say 200 over 120 (written 200/120), considerable attention should be given to reducing them. Some doctors feel a blood pressure reading over 160/110 requires treatment. High blood pressure should lead to a closer examination of the kidney function. Blood should be taken to be tested for cholesterol, sugar or uric acid (which could mean a tendency to gout). The doctor might ask for a chest x-ray to see if the heart is enlarged.

Pulse Rate: The pulse is taken at the wrist. The normal resting pulse ranges between 60 and 90 beats per minute. More rapid pulse rates may mean nervousness, fear or excitement. If you feel calm and your pulse rate is high, there is a possibility of anemia, infection, chronic illness of some kind, heart trouble or an overactive thyroid.[2] Only a doctor willing to sit and talk with you and evaluate your responses, however, can combine the symptoms and readings and differentiate one diagnosis from another.

Eyes: A quick glance at your eyes reveals to a practiced and alert doctor whether you have been drinking, are fatigued, have eyestrain or jaundice, are bruised from fighting or have eyes swollen from crying. Puffiness around the eyes might reveal kidney disease, low thyroid or that you are a candidate for plastic surgery. Dr. Isadore Rosenfeld in *The Complete Medical Examination* describes the method of eye testing, in which the doctor carefully feels around the eye to reveal the condition of the surrounding muscles.[3] Both eyelids are not always symmetrical, but if one or both are droopy, there may be cause for further concern. For patients over forty, a glaucoma check should be made each year.

Ears: By pulling the lobe of the ear, the doctor can see directly into the passageway to detect problems, if any, with the eardrum. The skin of the ear canal is subject to the same kinds of problems as the skin elsewhere on the body: eczema, infection and irritations. You might, at some time, have an infection in the skin of the ear canal, but it is hard to find since the spot changes color as the area is tensed by pulling.

Some kinds of hearing loss may be corrected by surgery, but damage related to the hearing nerves themselves may not be corrected by Western-type medical care. It is worth a try to have a treatment or two of acupuncture, now that it is available in the United States in many areas.

Circulatory System: If you have a problem with cold hands and/or feet, the doctor will probably check very carefully. As you get older, circulation problems generally increase and may involve your heart, your veins and arteries, or your thyroid.

Smoking has a very serious effect on some people, causing the blood supply to the extremities to diminish. If a person refuses to give up tobacco in any form, the pain may increase severely as the circulation becomes worse. There is even the possibility of losing a limb to Buerger's disease. Caffeine may also lead to vasoconstriction and cold extremities.

Breathing: Breathing processes must be automatic and regular, but variations in the breathing pattern can help spot arteriosclerosis, heart trouble or possible injuries to the brain.

Foul breath odor may indicate a long list of possible illnesses ranging from the use of drugs or tobacco to gangrene, diabetes, kidney disease or catarrh. Shortness of breath may signal the presence of edema, or fluids in the air passages.

Shallow breathing occurs in acute pulmonary disease. Asthmatic breathing has a kind of wheezing, harsh sound; bronchial breathing has a long, high-pitched sound when you exhale.

Chest Examination: The doctor checks for fluid in the lungs with the stethoscope, and detects early signs of heart failure, the wheezing of asthma, and the variable sounds of bronchitis. An electrocardiogram cannot be relied on to pick up heart murmur or the timid throb of a weak heart.

Breast Examination: The doctor will check both men and women for lumps in the breast. Women should not plan a visit to the doctor just before a menstrual period because the breasts fill up at that time and make it difficult for the doctor to examine the area properly. Some drugs may cause painful enlargements of the breast area, and men treated with female hormones for cancer of the prostate often have breast enlargement.

In the interest of keeping the number of x-rays one receives at a minimum, alternatives to the x-ray form of mammography should be considered. Xerography records the image on a selenium plate and produces a clear, detailed and immediately available picture. Another process, thermography, records the rise in temperature connected with injured tissue or multiplying cancer cells. Ultrasound is another alternative to x-ray. In this diagnostic procedure, sound waves pass through the body and their echoes are picked up on an electronic receiver. The echoes can outline a mass or tumor in the body, and can help distinguish between solid tumors and those filled with fluid such as cysts. Dr. Rosenfeld advises that x-ray should never be the only screening technique used in mammography.[4]

Heart Examination: A thorough physical examination, a carefully-taken history, and a list of your symptoms are of paramount importance in diagnosing heart troubles. The physician's judgment is supplemented by tests and instruments which give additional information about the heart's behavior. All tests require interpretation. Some are very sophisticated, others quite simple. For instance, you may be asked to do a measured amount of exercise, such as stepping up and down an abbreviated flight of stairs. The time it takes for your pulse rate to return to normal after such activity gives some indication of your heart's reserve capacity.

The heart is the center of the circulatory system of the entire body, and pumps blood throughout the system. The muscle itself has four chambers: two auricles and two ventricles, and is connected through the nervous system to the brain. Narrowed arteries make pumping blood to the extremities a problem, sometimes a painful one. But the pain might be a condition related to the tissue that wraps around the heart, called the pericardium, which can become infected with a virus. In many cases, these two conditions are difficult to distinguish from one another.

There is no such thing as a quiet heart. It is constantly clicking, lubbing and swishing, as its various parts take turns in regular or wavering rhythms. Heart murmurs, with their soft swishing or hissing sounds, are diagnosable with a stethoscope, but sometimes only after exercise and while you are lying on your left side on the examining table. Not all murmurs are significant; some come and go, but a murmur may indicate that blood is leaking back through an imperfectly closed valve. The fact that a child has a heart murmur is in itself no reason for a parent to be concerned or overanxious. Such murmurs may be heard in many normal children. As a matter of fact, about 30 percent of all normal healthy children have innocent heart murmurs at some time during their childhood. Sometimes these murmurs are heard only when a child is anemic or has an infection or fever.

Symptoms gathered by "hands-on" examination, plus use of the stethoscope and the electrocardiogram (EKG) *may* give some idea of the condition of your heart, but this is not certain. In general the EKG reveals heart problems only if you are having a heart attack at the time you are connected to the machine. This piece of equipment is used frequently in the doctor's office, and is of limited value. A new method of computer-oriented testing appears to be far more accurate than the EKG in detecting heart disease and analyzing results. Other sophisticated tests are available but they are expensive and may be more invasive.

Rectal Examination and Sigmoidoscopy: People often neglect to have this done, but it is necessary on a regular basis (especially in men over forty) to spot rectal and prostate cancer early. A rectal examination is performed by insertion of the physician's finger into the patient's rectum. The entire circumference of the lower bowel can be felt, allowing possible detection of cancer of the rectum. In the front portion of the rectum, the prostate gland can be palpated (touched, felt) and any suspicious hard areas that may indicate trouble can be felt.

Sometimes the doctor will decide to perform a sigmoidoscopy. The sigmoidoscope is a tube-shaped instrument, used to examine the lower sigmoid colon above the rectum.

You will be required to have an enema about an hour or two before the sigmoidoscopy. The position for examination is an odd one: You kneel on the examining table, buttocks skyward, with your head resting on the table, and trying not to notice the ridiculous position. The doctor will insert the instrument into the anus and examine the colon as far up as his instrument can extend.

Pelvic Examination: The pelvis is a bony structure that lies between the thighs and the trunk. Examination of the pelvic area is done to find problems in the female reproductive organs: the vagina, cervix, uterus, ovaries, or the bladder or rectum.

At the same time the pelvic examination is done, a Pap smear is usually taken to reveal the possibility of cancer in the cervix or uterus. The cervix is exposed by a vaginal speculum, an instrument that dilates (opens) the cavity to make the interior more easily visible. The opening of the cervix is scraped and material is taken from that area and from the top of the vagina and spread onto glass slides which are "fixed" immediately for later staining. The secretions contain many materials, including cells cast off by tissues of the area. Cancer cells in such preparations can usually be recognized by their response to special staining techniques. A presumptive diagnosis of cancer can be made from the early recognition of such cells.

Nevertheless, according to Dr. David M. Eddy, author of a study of cancer screening methods and techniques, the Pap smear a woman has had taken may be inaccurate unless the smear is taken properly.[5] Research shows that only 17 percent of general practitioners and 20 percent of gynecologists take Pap smears properly. Therefore, do not panic if the smear gives an unsatisfactory reading. A check on the accuracy of the reading, whether it was negative or positive, may be done in many communities by contacting the local Planned Parenthood Association and asking that they do a Pap smear for you. The cost is usually nominal, and you will be comforted by having a second opinion.

Nervous System Examination: The brain and its nerves, the spinal cord and its nerves, and the rest of the body's nerves are all interconnected. Together they comprise the entire nervous system. The nerves collect and send messages to the brain, so that the proper response is made. A good deal has been written about various aspects of the nervous system, because untreated high blood pressure is the major cause of brain hemorrhage and the most common reason for strokes of all kinds.[6]

Three mechanisms may cause stroke and brain damage: first, obstruction of the flow of the blood in one of the arteries; second, rupture of a blood vessel in the brain itself; and third, the movement of a blood clot (called an embolism) from another part of the body into the brain area. Problems in the elderly are often related to small, unrecognized strokes.

Signs of little strokes may appear before age forty. These do not invariably end in a catastrophic stroke, but they may indicate incipient or impending stroke. Small strokes give fair warning that preventive care is essential. People with TIAs (transient ischemic attacks—mini strokes) should see a physician immediately. Some of the warning signs are

—sudden temporary weakness or numbness of the face, arm or leg;
—temporary loss of speech or trouble in speaking or understanding speech;
—an episode of double vision;
—temporary dimness or loss of vision, particularly in just one eye;
—unexplained dizziness or unsteadiness, or momentary blackout;
—confusion or personality changes: previously stable and cheerful people may become irritable, sloppy, suspicious or behave in ways inconsistent with their previous life patterns.

These symptoms might indicate that parts of the brain may be affected by the insufficiency of blood. The parts can be identified by careful diagnosis.

Headaches and pain in the brain area deserve a great deal more attention than they get from most examining physicians. If headaches persist, make sure you get a good neurological examination!

Your doctor will test your reflexes with a special little rubber hammer to determine the level of coordination. Response to this slight tapping may vary from person to person, and there is no really "correct" amount of response, except that the response on both sides of the body should be fairly close.

General Physical Assessment: The doctor will probably do a general physical "overview" to spot physical abnormalities. Some requests may seem silly or simple, but can provide your doctor with important facts or insights. S/he will note how you stand and whether you can touch your nose with the finger of one hand and then the other with your eyes closed.

At this time your doctor may ask you to produce a sample of urine. In addition, you may go home with a little envelope containing something resembling a matchbook. As discussed earlier, instructions will accompany the kit. Two tiny samples of feces are to be added to each little circle of paper, one for each of two separate days. The booklet is then folded over, put into the accompanying envelope and sent to the doctor or directly to a laboratory. Examination of this matter may reveal data leading to various diagnoses. Don't fail to consult with your doctor about any findings.

The presence of problems in areas in which physicians have little exposure or training can be easily overlooked. For example, older people may too quickly be diagnosed as arthritic when the problem could instead be food allergy. Make sure you are given extensive tests before you accept a diagnosis of arthritis. You may also want to be tested for food allergy. Problems with diet as well as counseling for health education have fallen to nutritionists, homeopathic physicians and even to teachers in the public schools. In these cases, trust your instincts and feelings by alerting your doctor to areas and symptoms that you feel may have been overlooked.

Based on the examination, your doctor may make recommendations for care and treatment. In the event you do not feel well and ordinary tests have not revealed anything "significant," additional tests may be in order. To determine the presence of a toxic substance, an oversupply of copper, for instance, a more detailed and specialized type of testing must be done.

You will probably be given paperwork to bring to a laboratory and x-ray office with which your doctor is affiliated. Your examination is not over with yet. The next portion is done in the laboratory. Few definite conclusions can be drawn until the tests have been completed and the reports are given to the doctor.

Make sure you note all the information you can remember soon after leaving the doctor's office. You can use the following sample as a guide for recording data from any office visit.

Record of Doctor's Visit

Name of Patient _____

    Date:

    Hour in:

    Hour out:

Accompanied by_____

Symptoms described to doctor:

Examination procedures:

Diagnosis:

Medication Ordered:

Instructions: 1. Date of next visit:
             2. Lab tests required:
             3. Diet, exercise:

Comments:

NOTES

1. Isadore Rosenfeld, *A Second Opinion*, pp. 139–146.
2. Isadore Rosenfeld, *The Complete Medical Exam*, pp. 146–9.
3. Rosenfeld, *Complete Medical Exam*, p. 158.
4. Ibid., p. 99.
5. *Network News*, Newsletter of the National Women's Health Network, November/December 1982, p. 8.
6. Rosenfeld, *Complete Medical Exam*, p. 261.

4

Tests and More Tests

The laboratory work and x-rays you will have now are considered a normal extension of the "complete physical."

Your doctor's affiliation with a laboratory and radiology center (x-ray institution) will probably limit the places you may be able to go to have work done, as well as the kind of testing done. The first loyalty of most laboratories is to the referring doctor. It may be difficult to have results sent directly to you; if the doctor doesn't authorize it, the lab can't send you the results. However, it is mandatory in some states that you receive copies if you ask for them. Call your local Health Department to find out if your state is one in which the patient is entitled to receive such data directly. If not, you will have to get the results from your doctor's office.

Sometimes the physician maintains a laboratory of some sort in the office complex. While outside laboratories are supervised and monitored by the state and federal governments and the people working in them are required to be tested and licensed, the laboratory in the doctor's office is not under the same constraints. Sometimes untrained personnel may be doing the laboratory work and the results may not be accurate. The tests may even be misread.

Testing done at the laboratory usually will involve the taking of blood and a sample of urine unless the doctor has done this at the office. The most frequently ordered tests involve the analysis of urine and blood samples. However, additional tests such as feces, sputum and infection swabs for cultures may be requested by your physician in response to clues picked up in the interview as well as during the hands-on examination.

Urine Testing

Urinalysis: The normal color of urine is yellow to straw with some odor and a bitter saline taste. Eating certain foods—asparagus, for instance—may cause urine to have a characteristic odor and color. The colors deviating from normal may give some clues to diseases of various organs, or may indicate that a poison such as mercury or lead has been ingested.

Diabetes Testing: Urine is tested for the presence of glucose. Standards have changed for the diagnosis of diabetes and it is now known that even normal people may occasionally have traces of sugar in their urine. The actual testing is a fairly simple procedure and if the results warrant further investigation the doctor will recommend a glucose tolerance test of two to six hours duration.

The glucose tolerance test is also used to detect hypoglycemia or "low blood sugar." If low blood sugar is suspected, the solution is *not* more sugar. Additional supplies of sugar would put an undue strain on the body because the insulin-producing cells are already working too hard to deal with normal amounts of sugar.

In preparing for the glucose tolerance test, you will have to fast for eight to twelve hours prior to the testing. Then urine and blood samples are collected while your stomach is empty. A drink is then taken that contains 100 grams of glucose plus colors, flavorings and preservatives. A sample of urine and a sample of blood are taken thirty minutes later, and then every hour after that. This test may give results that suggest not only diabetes or hypoglycemia but possibly pancreas or endocrine problems.

The discomfort of having blood taken is the only physical inconvenience or pain of this testing procedure, but the boredom of sitting around for hours is often annoying. Be prepared and take along something to do.

Diabetes in children is a serious problem with a poor outlook for the future. In adults, however, late-onset diabetes often may be handled by adhering to a strict low-sugar, low-calorie diet. Patients may be put on oral medication but it has been determined that in many cases people do better on a strict dietary regimen than with medication.

Pregnancy Testing: At home, this test is performed by analyzing a urine sample. Done at the laboratory, blood or urine tests may be performed to confirm or deny results obtained at home.

Albumin and Globulin Test: When there is a question of infection in the liver and kidney area (with constipation, nausea and weakness as some of the symptoms) an albumin and globulin test is likely to be ordered. The globulins in the body are the immune bodies that fight diseases and carry some drugs, vitamins and hormones throughout the system. If albumin shows up in urine testing, it usually indicates kidney problems, but there is an exception: athletes may show small amounts of albumin in the urine after strenuous activity. This should disappear after a rest period, however.

Sometimes tests reveal too little albumin in the blood. When this occurs, the globulins may increase, indicating problems with the liver. When the globulins seem to be in greater supply, the liver has not been able to supply sufficient albumin to keep a balance.

Hematuria: This is a condition in which blood is detected easily in the urine and further examination and testing should follow. More likely, blood in the urine is only visible under a microscope. Don't panic. Blood in the urine is most commonly caused by a bladder infection. Menstruating women will occasionally have blood in the urine, as will those with kidney or bladder stones, nephritis, tumors or injuries; rarely due to inherited causes. Some types of tranquilizers and other medications could be responsible for this condition. Any drugs you are taking will show up on special analysis but some foods, like beets, may cause the urine to change color.

Many drugs damage the kidneys, whose function is to excrete these substances. Often when the offending drug is discontinued the kidneys return to proper functioning over a period of time.

Blood Tests

Complete Blood Count (CBC): Of all the tests done with samples of blood, probably the best-known is the one for hemoglobin (Hgb). In these tests, the red and white blood cells are counted, typed and examined under a microscope. The proportion of red and white cells indicates the possibility of disease, excessive blood loss or the inability to produce red blood cells as needed. Anemia is not a disease but a symptom of trouble, and a signpost that further analysis and examination are necessary. Don't stop at merely treating anemia. Find out the reason for the existence of the condition.

The function of hemoglobin is to circulate oxygen and remove carbon dioxide. The oxygen is taken to the lungs and released. Red blood cells contain hemoglobin and live about 120 days, then they are "recycled" into the yellow pigment called bilirubin. When your body can't tolerate a medication or when a poison is ingested accidentally, red blood cells are killed, sometimes faster than new cells can be created to take their place. At that time more bilirubin needs to be excreted than the body can handle and the "yellow" of the bilirubin shows up as jaundice. The same thing happens when the liver itself is "sick" and can't process the bilirubin sent to it.

The blood will reveal when the kidneys and liver are functioning. Both organs have many functions vital to the proper health of the body, so intensive testing should be done if there is any indication of a problem.

Cholesterol Testing: Despite the terrible things being said about cholesterol, it is a necessary ingredient for proper bodily functioning. Not only do we get cholesterol from the foods we eat, but the liver forms its own cholesterol. High cholesterol readings may be related to low thyroid functioning (metabolic disease), or to kidney disease as much as to the amount ingested in meals. A low cholesterol level could be related to starvation, an overactive thyroid, or an acute infection.[1]

Only a small number of people with high cholesterol suffer from heart attacks. There are conflicting reports about whether or not to lower cholesterol levels either through diet or drugs to protect people against heart attacks. There is not even any agreement about what is considered to be a "normal" amount of cholesterol in the blood.

Typically, doctors and medical researchers have tried to solve the problem of excessive accumulations of fatty tissue in the arteries by applying one drug or another, rather than intensively investigating the life habits of individuals with high, medium or low cholesterol and triglyceride levels. Perhaps the suggestion made by one doctor that cow's milk was never designed for human beings to drink should be researched further. Cows have three stomachs with which to digest; we have only one. Perhaps our bodies cannot digest cow's milk properly. In addition, some people are allergic to milk and milk products, and homogenized milk may cause congested veins and arteries.

Dr. Gerald Phillips of Columbia University published a study in the May 1983 issue of the *American Journal of Medicine* that seems to indicate that heart trouble has more to do with the level of female sex hormones in the body than with cholesterol. All people have both male and female hormones in their bodies, but people with "significantly high levels of estrogen" are the ones "least susceptible to heart disease," a term used to describe any pathological condition of the heart.[2]

Potassium Testing: Potassium balance with calcium and magnesium is essential for good muscle tone, especially for the heart muscles. It also plays a vital part in the proper function of nerve impulses.[3] If you are taking diuretics or high blood pressure medications, it is possible that the potassium in your body is being depleted. Too much potassium in the blood is indicative of possible heart and kidney failure. Checks should be done for potassium as people become older because of the relationship of this substance to the proper functioning of the heart.

Drugs can be prescribed to adjust the potassium level, but there are potential problems with using them. More satisfactory is the treatment of low potassium level by the addition of foods high in potassium such as citrus fruits, bananas, apricots, figs or peanuts.[4]

PKU: Testing for the condition of Phenylketonuria (PKU) in newborn babies is considered necessary to determine the ability of the patient to digest some proteins. This test is performed using blood samples. Many states require the blood of newborns to be tested in the hospital at birth.

The number of babies being born outside of hospitals is growing, so it has become a matter of urgency to inform mothers-to-be that their babies should be tested for PKU. PKU screening can discover those babies whose ability to digest some proteins is decreased or absent. This occurs in one child in every 20,000. Babies in whom this has been detected have been successfully treated, but those in whom it has not been found unfortunately have become retarded.

Even though PKU testing is done at birth, it is wise to repeat the test again in two to three weeks. If only one test is done, it is preferable to do the test two or three weeks after birth.

Urine tests are also available for PKU, but are not sensitive or conclusive enough and should not be taken as definitive.

Calcium and Phosphorous Testing: These two substances work together in the forming and strengthening of bones and other parts of the body in metabolism, in blood clotting, and in the transmission of nerve impulses. The adequacy of the calcium supply in the body is determined by a hormone secreted by the parathyroid gland which is behind the thyroid. When there is an overproduction of the parathyroid hormone, the calcium increases and the phosphorous decreases. When there is an underproduction of the parathyroid hormone, the opposite occurs.[5]

An oversupply of calcium in the blood may show up when too much vitamin D or milk is taken into the body, when too many antacids are consumed or even when the patient has hyperthyroidism.

A low blood calcium may indicate that not enough calcium is being ingested, that the parathyroid hormone is slowed down or inactive, that vitamin D cannot be absorbed in the body or is not available, or that the patient may have certain types of bone disease, such as rickets.

Abnormal calcium levels are indicative of a wide range of problems. Before conclusions can be reached, additional testing and even x-rays will have to be done.[6]

Thyroid Testing: Doctors often fail to do tests for thyroid dysfunction, although at one time it was suggested that alcoholics might have thyroid problems. Aside from clinical examinations, which often are not reliable, a number of laboratory tests are used to determine the quantities of the two thyroid hormones (T3 & T4) in the body. The results of these tests are influenced by iodides or drugs taken as long as six months before the thyroid testing is done. Therefore, careful documentation of previous examinations, such as x-rays or prescriptions, should be done before going ahead with the thyroid test, to rule out interference by iodine taken into the body in food or medicine.

If the test results are abnormal, most doctors believe the tests should be repeated before a diagnosis of thyroid dysfunction can be made. This problem is three times as common as PKU and newborn children should be tested for hypothyroidism that can cause mental retardation, nerve problems or stunted growth. Almost all states require such testing at the time of birth, but many do not enforce the law.

Note that the Pinckneys point out that the "protein-bound iodine test" is outmoded and that medical insurance programs may not be willing to reimburse you for the cost of this test.[7] They recommend the serum-free thyroxin (T4) as the most accurate single screening test for overall thyroid function.[8] A pituitary thyroid stimulating hormone test is also recommended.

Syphilis Testing: A Venereal Disease Research Laboratory (VDRL) test is usually required when people apply for a license to be married, no matter what their ages. Even older people, well past child-bearing age, could have syphilis. The VDRL test is also suggested when a skin disease fails to heal or when certain tropical diseases are suspected. Most states require that a woman have a VDRL when pregnancy is diagnosed.

Unfortunately, some of the types of testing done for venereal disease give false positive or false negative results; if one has a positive VDRL, a more specific test should be ordered, or at least a second and even a third VDRL test should be done. Some acute infections such as a smallpox vaccination may cause false positives.

Blood Typing: You might want to make a note of your "blood type," especially if you are a constant traveler, although blood given in an emergency transfusion is usually checked against your blood for compatibility before transfusion.

Other Tests

X-ray Testing: If x-ray testing is necessary, it may be done in the doctor's office, in an x-ray laboratory, in an office set up principally for this function or in the local hospital. Wherever it is done, the equipment should be in good repair, recently checked for accuracy, and operated by people trained in its use.

X-rays can penetrate many kinds of solid matter and make pictures on photographic emulsion that are black and white with some shades of grey. The rays emanating from the x-ray machine lower the ability of the body's immune system in its efforts to fight diseases. There have been many discussions in medical literature about limiting the amount of x-rays in an individual's lifetime as well as lowering the intensity of the rays.

In pneumonia cases, an x-ray shows whether the prescribed treatment is working. X-rays assist in the early detection of lung cancer, tuberculosis and other serious conditions. Discovering additional information from an x-ray, whether the view is frontal or from the side, is sometimes dependent upon whether you have been able to get old x-rays from your former physician, so that comparisons may be made of areas that appear to be presenting new problems. Old injuries may cause elderly people problems, and only by x-ray is this likely to be revealed. It is even possible that some pathological change has occurred at the site of a past break or injury.

For puzzling or more complicated cases, the new CAT-scan x-ray machinery is used. CAT stands for Computerized Axial Tomography, and consists of a "gantry" that has built into its circular opening the equipment that can take a picture of an entire section of the body, as if you were cut through at some point and examined. The bed upon which you rest may be rolled, so that any desired portion of the body or head can be made visible on the computer screen in the next room. Resting on the bed of the machine, you are slowly moved into the area of visibility, and the pictures are taken in sections one centimeter apart. Permanent x-ray films can be made from these views and may be kept for later comparison to show the progress of treatment.

Tuberculin Testing: A small injection is applied under the skin. In infected people, a redness or sore area is observed within forty-eight to ninety-six hours, but the tests do not reveal whether the tuberculosis sensitivity is showing up an active or an inactive infection. If you have recovered from a bout with tuberculosis, the test is likely to come up positive. In this case, x-ray examination should be done to establish whether the disease is still active.

Stool Samples: The sample may indicate trouble when it has a greyish or whitish glistening color. It may show fresh blood or have a tarry look, evidence of a hemorrhage condition. Samples that have a good deal of undigested food in them may indicate inflammation of the stomach and/or upper bowel.

Tarry-colored stools or stools with shreds of membrane or containing mucous may indicate conditions needing immediate attention. (See a medical dictionary for further discussion of these problems.)

Spirometry: Vital lung capacity is measured by inhaling as deeply as possible and blowing out as much air as possible into a machine called a spirometer. The quantity of expelled air varies with body size and age. Sometimes this test will be given to reveal breathing disorders, asthma, bronchitis or emphysema. It can also be used to monitor lung damage from environmental or industrial exposure to toxins and smoking. Some doctors will not test patients who continue to smoke. One doctor flatly stated, "I am not going to bother to heal you while you give me evidence you want to die by continuing to smoke."

The tests are complete when the doctor has reached a diagnosis. However, more tests may be done to monitor progress of the therapy. Reports on the tests done outside the office will be sent to the doctor, and either you will be told that there is no problem, or you will be asked to make an appointment to visit with the doctor again. If you don't telephone, you might not hear from the doctor at all, and you are left to assume that there is no problem. There are good reasons to check, however. There truly might be no problem, or the doctor may feel the problem is not serious enough to mention.

A warning is in order at this point: Often more tests are ordered than may be necessary. The more tests you have taken, the greater the possibility of a misdiagnosis. Poorly done tests and misreadings are more frequent than anyone would like to acknowledge.

In a reliable report of investigations of laboratories in one state whose results were tested for accuracy, a government survey found that *one test in every seven was in error or totally unreliable*. Multiplying that one out of seven by the number of tests taken in the United States per day, it is possible that at least one million tests per day, every day, are inaccurate. Some of them could be yours.

If all the previous testing has not provided enough results to offer the doctor a guide for establishing a diagnosis, you might be hospitalized for three or four days for additional testing. The rationale is that your diet—or fasting—can be better controlled in the hospital and you are available for testing when they are ready for you. You will find yourself donning a hospital gown that never quite meets at the back, eating bland foods, being awakened at unpredictable hours, submitting to being poked, bled, warmed, cooled, aspirated and frustrated, even though you are not in a real sense sick.

You will know the worst is over when the doctor comes in to discuss the results of the testing with you. The best thing to do is to get out your trusty pad and pen, and write down what you are told about what has been accomplished during your stay. Ask the name of the tests, including spelling of anything you hear that you don't understand, and ask what each was supposed to discover. Take down the information so that you can refer to it later.

The following procedures are advised: When a test seems to show abnormal results, have the test done *again* and a third time, if you want to be sure, *preferably at a different laboratory or office*, or *at the office of another physician*. Never rely on just one test result if the treatment designed for the condition requires surgery or serious and prolonged medication therapy. It is the job of the physician not only to diagnose the condition but to explain it to you. The doctor is also responsible for making clear why that particular test is being performed and what results s/he is seeking, *before you take the test*.

The Pinckneys warn that between 25 and 50 percent of the tests that turn out to be abnormal are not reported by the doctor to the patient. It is important that you get your own copy of the test results, and learn to compare it to the "norms."

In many states, the doctor is required to let you know the names of the tests you are being asked to take. If a request to the doctor or the doctor's office fails to produce copies of the test results, you may obtain a subpoena (a court order) to get the data you want and are entitled to.

Diagnostic laboratory tests are based upon a number of different principles. In infectious diseases, the tests ordinarily depend upon finding and identifying the germs that cause the particular disease. In diseases of the blood, the tests are based upon direct microscopic examination of the blood cells and counting the different types of cells in a measured quantity of blood, in either case comparing the results with the normal. In cancer, the diagnostic procedure is based upon microscopic examination of a bit of tissue removed from a suspicious lump or ulcer.

Some blood analysis may have to be done in the event the doctor is planning to give you medication. More thorough exploration of the obvious tests, more intensive than the ones done in the doctor's office or the laboratory may need to be done in a hospital. It is hoped that these tests will reveal additional information. Conditions that could and should have been detected much earlier can develop into illnesses and diseases that could stay with you for the rest of your life. The "If I thought you needed it, I would have done it" response by the doctor does not assure you of adequate testing. In the final analysis it is your life, and if you want to live it at peak zest, it is up to you to make sure that whoever is ordering and doing the testing is doing an adequate job.

Some of the tests, such as the six-hour glucose tolerance test, take a long time to complete and are often omitted entirely from the testing procedure unless you insist. There might be so few positive results from testing people for a particular routine that doctors omit it. There is no way to determine whether that lengthy test or that annoyingly complicated one is going to indicate what is wrong with you when you don't feel well and nothing has surfaced as an explanation.

In the event you feel doctors have been trying to treat your symptoms for years rather than determining the actual cause of your problems, it might be well for you to request additional laboratory testing. Allergy testings also may be requested to establish sensitivity to foods that children or adults cannot tolerate. These allergy tests reveal that certain foods can produce reactions which seem to have mental and behavioral symptoms. Although many doctors habitually order an excessive number of tests, it is not contradictory to advise additional testing when necessary.

Many doctors claim they "over-test" in order to protect themselves against malpractice suits. However, excessive testing is costly to the patient— monetarily, physically and emotionally. Patients tend to sue their doctors when they have been treated with a poor attitude. In the courtroom, many patients accuse the doctor of refusing to discuss the diagnosis, medication or treatment with them. Often patients state that their doctor was unwilling to entertain the possibility of an alternative diagnosis.

NOTES

1. Cathey Pinckney and Edward R. Pinckney, *Encyclopedia of Medical Tests.* pp. 309–10.
2. *American Journal of Medicine,* vol. 74, no. 5, May 1983, pp. 863–9.
3. *Taber's Cyclopedic Dictionary,* 14th edition, p. 1144.
4. Joe Graedon, *The People's Pharmacy,* p. 266.
5. Pinckney and Pinckney, *Patient's Guide to Medical Tests,* pp. 42–43.
6. Ibid., p. 43.
7. Ibid., p. 264.
8. Ibid., p. 264.

5

Patients' Rights and Responsibilities

Medical professionals in all medical settings—solo practices, group practices, local health centers, hospitals and long-term institutions—are required to recognize the code of Patients' Rights.

Often when you enter an institution you are given a copy of the Patients' Rights code. A framed copy of the document may be hung on the wall in the doctor's office where you can read it while you wait. In case of emergency when the patient is not conscious, either through accident or illness, a relative is usually given a paper detailing the patient's rights. It is expected that, when possible, the relative will share this information with the patient.

As a patient you have the legal right:

—to informed participation in all decisions involving your health care program;

—to privacy regarding the source of payment for treatment and care. This also includes access to a full range of available forms of treatment, without regard to the source of payment for that treatment or care;

—to prompt attention, especially in an emergency;

—to a clear explanation of all procedures. This includes an explanation of all possible risks and side-effects of such treatment or procedures. You will not be expected to undergo such treatment or operation without a thorough understanding and stipulation. All of the explanations offered should be incorporated into the consent form for you to sign;[1]

—to be informed of the right to refuse any test or procedure designed for the education of medical personnel rather than for your own direct personal benefit;

—to refuse any particular drug, test or procedure offered for your care. If you have not given consent, you may refuse to take whatever is offered. It will then be the responsibility of the hospital, the nurses or your lawyer to communicate with the doctor and ask that the treatment be discussed with you. You should feel confident the treatment is in accordance with your mutual understanding with your doctor. This includes surgical procedures as well. Mechanical restraints, hot or cold baths, or medication by mouth or hypodermic may not be used over your objection;

—to be treated with respect and dignity; to have privacy not only in regard to your person, but also regarding information imparted to the hospital staff, other doctors, residents, interns, medical students, researchers, nurses and other patients;

—to leave the health care facility regardless of your physical condition or financial status, although you may be requested to sign a release stating that you are leaving against the medical judgment of the doctor or the hospital.[2]

For those patients who are in a long-term care facility such as a nursing home or state institution, the following rights are particularly pertinent, although they apply to patients in any kind of facility as well:

—to receive and send sealed mail;

—to make and receive telephone calls;

—to receive visitors of your own choosing during visiting hours, including physicians and clergymen.

In addition, if you are hospitalized for nervous and mental disorders, whether voluntarily or involuntarily, there is an obligation to give you a physical examination within a reasonable length of time and to establish a treatment plan appropriate for the disorder diagnosed. Facilities do differ from state to state, however, and the time between admission and examination may vary slightly. It is mandatory that the examination be done and that suitable treatment be made available.

Minors may be treated for alcoholism, drug dependency, or venereal disease without the knowledge or consent of a parent or guardian. In some states, too, communication between a student and teacher regarding alcohol and drug-related therapies cannot be required to be disclosed; such interchanges are treated as confidential. In these cases the teacher or advisor cannot be held liable concerning this confidential information.

A large percentage of people at the poverty level are young women with children. The availability of health care for them and their children has become a source of hardship. Made helpless by interminable waits, expensive medication, and too little effort on the part of health care personnel to give sufficient attention to what could be complicated or multiple problems, many despair. If a woman in this situation becomes "demanding," she may be ignored or maltreated. She may not even realize that sometimes clinic care is more expensive than private care received from a general practitioner or a specialist at a smaller hospital.[3] Actually, people who go to clinics are doing the health personnel a favor, since teaching hospitals "need" patients in order to teach medical professionals and to give them experience they would find difficult to get otherwise.[4]

If you feel you have not been treated fairly, ombudsmen, or patient advocates, are often available as part of the hospital staff. Trained to be diplomatic, caring, and concerned, they will make every effort to take a complaint to the proper authorities, and hopefully, the problem will be resolved. If it is not settled, your lawyer or the local Legal Aid Society also will make an attempt to resolve the situation.

The doctor is obliged to respond to your questions about the course of treatment, the outlook for recovery, and the statistical effectiveness of the proposed treatment. You have the right to know the percentage of successful conclusions the proposed therapy has produced. It is *your* decision to make. People who learn that 50 percent of the suggested treatments were effective must weigh the options carefully. Expect your doctor to be able to present alternatives to the suggested treatment if at all possible.

In most states you, or someone responsible for you, have the right to review medical records and to get copies of them. Sometimes the doctor or the hospital is reluctant to turn over records or allow them to be reviewed. However, in most states there are statutes that permit a judge to order the doctor or hospital to produce all the data they have regarding a patient at the written request of the patient or the interested relative. There is no penalty in many states when a hospital forces a person to the expense, time and effort of going to court to secure release of data. Usually nothing can be done if the hospital will only consent to send a copy rather than the original of the records, even if the original is required for litigation. However, it is not necessary to be in litigation to see your medical or hospital records. Just wanting to see them is sufficient, and they must be made available for viewing when a written request is made.

There are exceptions. If the doctor or the hospital determines that it is not in your best interest to give you access to your records, they may withhold them. In that case, it would be necessary for you or your guardian to consult a lawyer.

No information of any nature regarding you may be given out to people who telephone or come in person to inquire, if you have expressly refused to permit it. All you must do is provide a written order to your doctor, to the hospital, or to any treatment center in which you have been seen, stating that you don't want any information given out about you. Until and unless you give a written order, though, the hospital or doctor may give out your name, admit the fact that you are a patient, and state your general condition.

There is always a problem with medical records that affect other people, when disclosure might do harm to others. This would be considered sufficient reason to withhold medical records.

Evidence that you, or someone responsible for your well-being, has been informed about the procedures is based upon what is currently being debated as "informed consent." How thoroughly a patient is briefed regarding the hazards of certain types of medication or the seriousness of a particular operation, is dependent upon the physician. Court cases, however, do seem to reveal that patients and their relatives are not happy with the amount of factual and statistical information being revealed at the time of "consent." Read the consent form carefully, and ask that any vague or technical terms be explained. You have the right and privilege to cross out or alter anything that appears on the consent form. You need only ink in your initials above or near the alteration to indicate that you did it yourself and were aware of what you were causing to have altered. For instance, if you are being examined for a possible malignancy in the breast, you might want to reserve the right to choose whether to have the entire breast and surrounding lymph glands removed, or have a lumpectomy (removal of the lump only) instead. You have no choice if you have signed the traditional consent form, because if it has not been altered it gives the doctor the sole right to make the decision.

The consent form, except in the case of emergency, could and should be available to you for examination and discussion either with your doctor, an advisor or a lawyer *before* you enter the hospital for the planned operation. The hustle and bustle of a hospital admission, with its shuffling of papers and identification of insurance forms, does not give sufficient recognition to the fact that the consent form is also a legal document, deserving of the most profound and searching examination of its wording—and re-wording, if desired or necessary. If you take the time and effort to examine what you are consenting to, you won't find yourself planning to have a D & C (dilation and curettage: a scraping of the wall of the uterus) and coming out of the anesthetic to discover you have had a hysterectomy.

Some in the medical profession feel that a greater use of "informed consent" would solve the problem of malpractice. Instead of fighting the idea, as they have in the past, doctors could accept it, embrace it and, in fact, give the patient the entire story about the risks and the alternatives to the treatment. Then the patient could share the decision about which direction the treatment should take.

Doctors have consistently ignored the signals coming from the self-care movement, according to Drs. Pellegrino and Thomasma.[5] They also note that doctors have continued to ignore alternative medical systems to their own detriment.

More and more people are articulating their apprehensions that recommended procedures are not in their best interests. They are being required to take on faith too many questionable procedures. The image and myth of the doctor as humanitarian, presented to the American public for so long, often doesn't fit the reality of the physicians we encounter who seem cold and money-centered.[6]

There are still problems in the definition of "doctoring" that need to be clarified. For example, some children attending school need medication during the time they are away from home and away from the jurisdiction of parents or guardians. Teachers, with their effective unions, have in many instances defended their right to refuse to be held responsible for what could be a touchy issue: the timing of medication which might affect either its effectiveness or the behavior of the child in the classroom, the amount of the dosage, over which a teacher most certainly should have no control, and the reporting of effectiveness of the therapy. In a classroom of fifteen to thirty children, this concentration on one or two children could seriously interfere with teaching.

Too often the responsibility for dispensing medication to a student has been given to unwilling and busy office personnel. While answering the telephone and attending to the needs of the principal or teachers, they may reach for medication belonging to one or another of the children lined up on the benches in the office. With no union defending their right to refuse this imposition, office workers do the best they can, but warily and with just cause. In today's budget crunch, school nurses are few and far between.

Another problem is related to alternative forms of therapy such as acupuncture. The efficacy of acupuncture can be denied only by those people who refuse to see. The right to seek acupuncture treatments has finally been upheld where doctors had previously charged the practitioners with practicing medicine without a license. The doctors contended that anything that punctured the skin was within their jurisdiction, and a practitioner of acupuncture had to have a medical license. The court found that forcing acupuncturists to have medical licenses limited access for people choosing that form of treatment. Since few doctors were trained in either the theory or practice of acupuncture, the medical license restriction interfered with the right of individuals to choose the form of treatment they preferred.

As was pointed out: "The administration of licensing laws is carried out in ways that reduce the dissemination of information. By granting physicians a monopoly on health care services the laws provide no incentive for physicians to inform people."[7]

The question was raised as to whether doctors legally should be the sole purveyors of health care services in such fields as nutrition, prevention of illness, and sex therapy. In these areas, doctors often have had little training and are less competent than the practitioners of the alternative forms of therapy they are working so hard to suppress with legislation. If the situation and statistics were presented more carefully, it would be found that misdiagnoses—as well as some of the dangerous techniques and treatments prescribed—create the situation in which a doctor, with a tendency to overtreat, may do patients more harm than good. Some studies show that alternative health care practitioners provide safer services than do physicians.[8]

The present medical licensing laws forbidding anyone without a medical license from offering health care advice, diagnosis, treatment, or preventive services could rule out the publication of newspaper items and columns, the work of laboratory technicians, research scientists, and mutual aid groups which assist people who suffer from chronic ailments.

The expected glut of physicians in the near future will intensify the problems of winning the right to alternative therapies, and the right of practitioners to set up such practices. Because of their wealth, doctors are able to battle for legislation that will not necessarily improve our health system, but will protect their incomes. Witness the millions of dollars spent in 1984 by doctors in Florida to push for legislation to limit the amount of money that can be awarded in malpractice suits—without any accompanying promise to clean their houses of the incompetent doctors in their ranks.

Knowing your rights and claiming those rights are two entirely different situations. Patients have found that questioning diagnoses or treatment methods has often resulted in the doctor's withholding of vital information. It has become the custom in some areas for a friend to accompany a patient into the doctor's examining room. You should feel comfortable with your doctor's response to your concerns, especially since when you choose a doctor, you almost inevitably choose potential hospital care as well.[9] In some way, doctors seem to feel personally threatened when they can't find a physical cause for symptoms you report. This can lead them to label your illness "psychosomatic" when there is no evidence of psychological symptoms. In some cases, the doctor isn't even qualified to diagnose in the psychological or psychiatric field.[10]

Unless the right to disagree or challenge is firmly established in health care, the doctor may not recognize your right to know. Don't retreat! Demand an explanation in simple, understandable language, even over the plaintive "What's the matter, don't you trust me?"[11]

A grass-roots organization is springing to life in the United States, in an attempt to share knowledge of physicians' competence and willingness to be open about health information, treatments, fees, and alternative forms of therapy. Based in Emmaus, Pennsylvania, the organization is called People's Medical Society. They have established a "Code of Practice" which they have sent to doctors and asked them to follow. The code is an attempt to expand the hard-won rights of patients, and at least one doctor in each of thirty states has agreed to live by it.

The code provides for printed scheduling of fees for office visits, testing and surgery; scheduling of hours during each week when the physician will be available for telephone consultation; scheduling sufficient time for each patient; permitting a friend or relative in the examination room; providing copies of test results; discussing fully the diagnosis and prognosis;

suggesting alternative forms of therapy whenever possible; describing his/her own qualifications for performing the recommended therapy; informing the patient of support groups and publications that will help the patient understand and monitor his/her problem; and proceeding with treatment only when the patient understands the benefits and risks in the chosen treatment.[12]

This is a step in the right direction. Enlargement of this movement could lead to a greater effort toward preventive medicine, as well as toward thoughtful, careful treatment of those already ill.

In order to convince doctors that patients can be treated as intelligent and responsive individuals, you as a patient must be responsible and cooperative and carry out your share of a recuperation program. You must have a share in working toward the solution. To this end, be prepared to arrive on time for appointments, to talk honestly about medication you are taking, to willingly discuss your symptoms, family and former medical history, to discuss your fears and reservations regarding the doctor's care, the form of treatment and the medication prescribed. In this way, your doctor can deal with your concerns. A physician can't answer questions you haven't asked, and can't explain away your apprehensions if you haven't discussed them.

Be sure to take only the amount and kind of medication your doctor orders to give the treatment a chance to work. Too often, people feel that if one pill is good, two or three will be even better. They may then end up with side effects that could have been predicted if discussed with the doctor. On the other hand, not taking the medication at all, or stopping too soon, will not give the doctor the opportunity to assess the value of the treatment. Don't fail, if at all possible, to let the doctor know when you are feeling better and no longer need treatment. Hearing from you will help the doctor evaluate the therapy ordered.

Last but not least, unless you have one of the rare doctors who will wait for Medicare or Medicaid reimbursement, pay your bill.

Yes, patients are requiring a much higher standard of care and better service than they did ten years ago. However, we are all past, present, and future consumers of health care and it makes good sense for us to organize and define our goals so that we may plan for more humane, cooperative and intelligent medical attention—while we are healthy.

NOTES

1. Boston Women's Health Collective; *Our Bodies, Ourselves* p. 356.
2. Ibid., p. 356.
3. Ibid., p. 358.
4. Ibid., p. 358.
5. *Mother Jones*, vol. 5 no. 7, June, 1982, p. 49.
6. *Our Bodies, Ourselves*, p. 358.
7. Lori B. Andrews, *Deregulating Doctoring*, p. 13.
8. Ibid., p. 4.
9. *Our Bodies, Ourselves*, p. 358.
10. Ibid., p. 349.
11. Ibid., pp. 349–51.
12. People's Medical Society, *Code of Practice*.

6

A Second Opinion

There is usually more than one way to treat your ailments, although you may not be aware of the alternatives. Doctors are supposed to discuss them with you, but they rarely do.

Usually the methods used for diagnosis are simple, painless and not intrusive. However, in a growing number of cases, the methods of diagnosis have grown increasingly intrusive—and sometimes dangerous. Among the most dangerous tools in a physician's or dentist's office is the x-ray or fluoroscope machine. These can produce cancer in you or leukemia in your unborn child. Don't underestimate the lethal potential of this "most misused of medical tools," just because it is heavily used in the treatment of cancer.[1] The damaging results of other intrusive diagnostic techniques can be seen even more quickly than x-ray, whose effects may not even show up for twenty years. "Catheterization kills one in fifty people. . . and there is no evidence that its results extend either the life expectancy or the comfort of the patient."[2] When several tests are given at once, and material is swallowed, injected or applied, the combinations often are distressing to the patient and color the results as well.

When tests are embarrassing, uncomfortable, or expensive, people will delay as long as possible before making an appointment with the doctor. Of course this delay may not be healthy and may make further testing necessary.

In situations where there is the possibility of major surgery, where an illness is diagnosed as very serious, or when the patient is being treated for a condition and the treatment doesn't seem to be helping, it may be time for another medical opinion.

You might worry that your doctor has a tender ego and will react strongly to your suggestion that another doctor be consulted. You might be afraid of offending your doctor by asking for a second opinion, or of not being treated well by the doctor in the future.

Not all doctors are conscientious about keeping up to date in their field. Although they may know about new methods as reported by highly reputable colleagues or journals, they are under no obligation to apply this knowledge. Sometimes they refuse to do so.[3]

If your doctor is not keeping up with the latest information in the field, perhaps you ought to change doctors anyway. The newspaper, radio, and television are constantly bringing to public attention the newest advances in many fields, in addition to magazines which devote pages to the subject of health problems. You would be justifiably apprehensive with a doctor who hadn't heard of a method of treatment you heard about, since discussion in the medical journals should have elaborated on this subject long before it became available to the general public.

If you think your doctor would be offended if you suggested consulting another physician for a second opinion, proceed carefully. In such a case, you might decide to change doctors. If you do, *write* a request that your medical records be sent to your new physician. The doctor is required to do so.

On the other hand, try giving the doctor the opportunity to discuss working with a consultant. Your doctor might welcome the opportunity to share the responsibility for determining the diagnosis and treatment of a serious or difficult problem.

Not only do doctors disagree about the methods of treating a particular illness, but they also may disagree on the diagnosis, the prognosis, and even the ability of the patient to handle the ramifications of an honest opinion about the entire condition.

An organization called PRESSO (Program for Elective Surgical Second Opinion) sponsored by Blue Cross/Blue Shield of Greater New York, is growing, which not only expresses an opinion about diagnosis and therapy, but also provides the names of at least two near-by board-certified specialists in the field. You choose the doctor for the second opinion and if you want to, you may use the second name offered for a third opinion. Your medical information is sent by PRESSO to the specialist you have chosen to consult, and the second doctor has the data to study before you arrive for your examination.

The list of consultants is compiled with the agreement that they will remain consultants, will not treat you or operate on you, and will accept a set fee for consultation.

The doctors in the PRESSO program have reported a new cooperation between doctor and patient, as well as an awareness of alternative forms of therapy. They state there is a new climate of question-and-answer evolving in the doctor's office by intelligent and alert patients. The very existence of a second-opinion program seems to prompt a more conservative and careful opinion from the doctors consulted first. Eventually, only about half the patients asked for a second opinion, and it was estimated that there was a saving of $3 to $4 for every dollar spent on medical care, with a 20 percent drop in surgery.[4]

Without a chapter of PRESSO nearby, there are still effective ways to get a second opinion:

—Ask your doctor to suggest a consultant. You may be given a name of an individual with whom your doctor works well.

—Choose a consultant yourself, either by using the *Directory of Medical Specialists* or through the recommendation of a friend or family member. Discuss your choice with your doctor. If your doctor has never worked with a consultant before, s/he might welcome the opportunity to do so. In either of these cases, send a copy of your records out before you visit so the consultant will be aware of the areas of controversy.

—Choose another doctor on your own and have a consultation without revealing the fact that you have had previous attention to the problem. Choose, if you can, to go to another community or area, served by another hospital or laboratory, if new tests or x-rays will need to be done.

Dr. Isadore Rosenfeld, in his book *Second Opinion*, points out that there are people who shop for diagnoses until they get one that suits their fancy.[5] This could be dangerous. You could spend the time during which something could be done to alleviate a condition just waiting for opinion after opinion, until you have reached a point of no return.

If the condition is considered life-threatening, do rely on the considered opinion of your doctors. Don't delay unnecessarily.

If your condition is not life-threatening but chronic, and you feel that little or no progress is being made, read on. Researching on your own is probably the answer.

NOTES

1. Robert S. Mendelsohn, *Male Practice*, p. 50.
2. Ivan Illich, *Medical Nemesis*, p. 94.
3. Boston Women's Health Collective, *Our Bodies, Ourselves*, p. 361.
4. Mark Schacter, "Evaluation of a Surgical Second Opinion Program," in QRB, January 1983 vol. 9 no. 1, p. 11.
5. Isadore Rosenfeld, *A Second Opinion*, p. 28.

7

Medications

Many patients want a prescription to last until the next planned visit to the doctor. In that case the doctor will send you out with one, and perhaps even two, three, or four prescriptions in your hand. All patients do not feel this way, however. Some even refuse to take a prescribed drug until they look it up in the *Physician's Desk Reference* or another reference book.

Do not fail to let the doctor know from the start if you do not like to take medication, so that this can be entered on your chart right in the front. Studies show that large numbers of patients don't take the medicines ordered for them. The sale of books listing medicines that don't work such as *How to Be Your Own Doctor—Sometimes* and *Pills That Don't Work* indicate that the time of patients automatically taking medications without question is coming to a close. Studies also reveal that when people do not get a full description of what the doctor feels is wrong, including an explanation of what the drug is supposed to do, frequently they just don't take it.

This is especially true of older people. The media has helped to confirm their feeling that they have been getting an overload of medications, and they have been building an inner warning system. They examine quite carefully what they are ordered to take and consult each other about it. Then they often conclude they either did not need this particular drug or did not need any drug. They also may challenge the dosage prescribed. Many express apprehension regarding foods or liquids that should or should not be taken while using prescribed medication, and are angry that these limitations were not discussed with them.

Other people worry that medication they are being urged to take could make them unable to drive even if an emergency occurred and their help was desperately needed. Many elderly also have reservations that some drugs don't work well together, are too harsh, or are not suitable for their needs.

Drowsiness at an inappropriate time, unexpected impotence, itching in areas that cannot easily be reached, and queasiness can make an individual wary not only of the medication ordered this time, but also of future prescriptions.

There is no reason not to ask the doctor about the prescription at the time it is offered. Insist upon a full disclosure. When you get home and start to take the drugs, and find that problems turn up, telephone the doctor's office. Insist upon speaking to the doctor directly. Don't settle for a secretary or nurse. Only the doctor can prescribe a substitute medication, if a substitute is necessary.

According to Dr. Ivan Illich, dependence on drugs and tranquilizers has risen 290 percent since 1962—a period during which per capita consumption of liquor rose by only 23 percent and the estimated consumption of illegal opiates increased by about 50 percent.[1] Profits to the drug companies are phenomenal: markups of 140 times the cost of producing the drugs are not unusual.[2] Increasingly, Illich states, doctors work with two groups of addicts: people for whom they have prescribed medications who have become addicted to their medicines, and those who suffer from the consequences of their prescriptions with failing bodies and weakened minds. The richer the community, Dr. Illich contends, the larger the percentage of patients who belong in both categories.[3]

Over-prescribing drugs has become all too common. Antibiotics, for instance, are the most commonly over-prescribed drugs, often recommended by doctors for colds, flu, and other illness for which they are not effective. In addition, many people are sensitive to antibiotics and may develop other problems, such as vomiting, diarrhea, and yeast infections, while taking them. Most important, bacteria can build up a resistance to antibiotics so that a person who has frequently taken them for minor ailments may find them ineffective for something serious.

If the doctor offers a prescription, be sure to discuss any medication you are already taking. Mention food supplements, aspirin, diuretics, laxatives, and vitamins. Refer to the list you brought with you.

Ask your doctor to prescribe your medication generically whenever possible. The word generic refers to a general classification. Generic drugs are identified by their chemical compounds, not by pharmaceutical companies' trade names, and are far less expensive than brand name products.

Examine the prescription after it has been written. Ask the doctor to pronounce the name of it, if you can't read or pronounce it. Ask for the correct spelling.

Don't hesitate to ask what the medication is supposed to do. Often the only thing a doctor knows about the prescribed drugs is what the drug company's representative has said and s/he might not even be clear about that. If your doctor doesn't know anything about a medication *don't take it*.

Pharmaceutical companies subsidize the curricula of the medical schools. They donate drugs, endow chairs, and send representatives to the medical schools on a regular basis to familiarize interns with their products early on. Huge amounts of money are spent yearly to induce physicians to prescribe their brand-name drugs[4], so you can assume that your doctor is not going to prescribe dandelion greens or yogurt.

Too often when the salesperson comes for a visit, the doctor is in a hurry. The pharmaceutical representative finds that time does not permit discussion of details about the products being recommended. Confusion may result. Feeling adequately informed, the doctor may not read the slip enclosed with the package of medication that warns about who should and should not take it and specifies the side-effects.

More frightening is the fact that some doctors are being paid an average of $35,000, and a few as much as $1,000,000 a year, to experiment with medications on their patients to see whether animal "tolerance" results are similar to "tolerance" in human beings.[5] Doctors are required to get a consent form from a patient before using experimental drugs.

A patient in New York City was treated for a severe case of arthritis with an experimental drug that had been cleared for use upon humans. Instead of monitoring the patient carefully, the doctor went to Europe on vacation. By the time the doctor returned, the patient's liver had been fatally damaged by the drug, and there was no way she could be saved. She died shortly after his return.[6]

The Food and Drug Administration (FDA) maintains a list of doctors currently testing drugs on human subjects, or who have in the past tested drugs on their patients. Death of a patient taking an experimental drug must be reported. When the death of the New York patient was investigated, the FDA agents noted in the report that until several days before her hospitalization and death, her charts indicated that she was doing "normally" well. They were puzzled.

Examining the clinical reports more closely, they discovered the doctor was out of the country when the medication was administered. The reports signed by the doctor failed to reflect the fact that he was not taking care of the patient at all. If the patient had not died, millions of people with arthritis could have been exposed to the same fate before the evidence was sufficiently damaging for the FDA to order the medication removed from the market.

One physician expressed the view that falsified studies are regularly slipping through the FDA screening processes. In these cases, affluent and influential companies are pursuing financial reward rather than drug safety with regularity. This physician feels that fraud and outright alteration of data is done by some pharmaceutical companies and in some instances is overlooked by prominent physicians.[7]

Be very careful about the medication your doctor orders for you. You should investigate whether this particular medicine should be taken before certain tests are made. Some drugs *must not* be ordered for *any* patient before certain tests are performed. For instance, one drug should not be given to patients who are anemic, who have high blood pressure, or thyroid dysfunction. Yet one doctor, without any kind of tests whatever, prescribed it for me as "a muscle relaxant." Checking, for me, is a standard procedure and in this case I read the entry in the *Physician's Desk Reference (PDR)* with special interest. This medication could have caused aplastic anemia (failure of the bone marrow to produce red blood cells).

If you hunt in your nearby public library, you might be able to find a recent copy of *Physician's Desk Reference*, published by Medical Economics Company of Oradell, New Jersey. Keep in mind that the *PDR* relies on information produced by the drug companies; it is neither unbiased nor complete. This book comes out every year, with occasional supplements published during the year. Consult the most recent issue you can locate, but not one that is more than two years old if possible. If it is not available on the open shelves of the public or medical library, ask the librarian for it. You will probably have to sign it out and may only be permitted to use it for a limited period of time.

The *PDR* contains five indexes described below, at least one of which will enable you to find the information you want about the medication that has been ordered for you.

1. Manufacturer's index—contains the address and emergency telephone number of the firm that made the medication. They may be called any time.

2. Product name index—lists the name of the medication as it is offered on the market. The list is in alphabetical order and contains page numbers that will permit you to go right to the information you want.

3. Product classification index—groups medications into categories and also includes page numbers.

4. Generic and chemical name index—lists the medications under the headings of their principal ingredients.

5. Product identification index—presents color pictures and shows the actual size of one dose of each drug. If you don't have the name of the product or the name of the company, having one of the pills will make it possible for you to identify it.

On the appropriate page there will be a description of the medicine, a list of its ingredients, a warning about who should not be taking it, whether it should be monitored closely or not at all, and a list of the side-effects that might be encountered. These data are usually a reproduction of the slip enclosed with the medication when a bottle or carton is bought at the pharmacy. Too few people realize the importance of reading carefully the slip that comes with their medicine and of retaining it for future reference.

If you don't have the slip that should have come with the medication, make a copy from the *PDR*. If small quantities of the medication were prescribed for you, it may have been dispensed without the manufacturer's descriptive literature being enclosed. Take a trip to the nearest *PDR* and check it out.

If your medication is not listed in the *PDR*, it is either very new and has not yet been listed, or is an experimental drug. If it is very new, it might be listed in the supplement. The librarian may have tucked this into the back pocket of the book.

If the drug you are researching is experimental, you have the right to discuss with the doctor the possible risks involved in taking an untried medicine. Insist that it is your decision—not the doctor's—to decide whether to take the chance. The discussion should include data on where, when, and under whose auspices this drug was proved usable on animals, and certified copies of the test results should be available for your records. Side effects are bound to be different when a human being uses the medication, so monitoring is of vital importance. As soon as you realize you are taking an experimental drug, set up a schedule that will provide sufficient supervision, as well as a method of communicating directly with the doctor in the event of an emergency.

On the last page and on the back cover, the *PDR* has a two-page description of how to handle drug overdoses. It is written in medical terminology, so other helpful materials should be available in your household for emergency reference.

Now your notebook of collected data will come in handy again. Don't fail to turn to the first index and take down the full name, address, and emergency telephone number of the company that makes the medication you are taking. If you have side-effects from the medication, check with your doctor first. If your doctor is not available, don't hesitate to call the pharmaceutical company. Be prepared to tell them the details about the side-effects you are experiencing, where you bought the medication, the name, address, and telephone number of the doctor who prescribed it, the date it was purchased, how many pills were ordered and how often you were supposed to take them. They will want to know how many you have already taken and when the symptoms or side-effects started to occur.

If your doctor insists you take the medication even with the side effects, read the material from the *PDR* again, then tell the doctor you plan to discuss the matter with a friend or your lawyer if necessary. Think this through carefully, then *make your own decision and stick with it*.

Count the number of pills dispensed to you. See if it tallies with the number ordered on the prescription. Costs are high and you want what you have paid for. If the doctor has prescribed a large quantity of pills, ask whether you will be free of your problem at the end of the dosage. Find out how long you should expect to take the medication before you see some results.

If you have taken the pills before and they have not given you any problems, examine the new batch before using them. Make sure they seem to be the same as the ones previously supplied to you. Sometimes pharmaceutical firms change the ingredients or the bases of pills without notice. Different formulas can create allergic reactions or side-effects in some people.

If you are travelling, make a photostat of your prescription to take along, even if you take the pills with you. You might stay longer than expected, or have reactions to the pills after you have reached a new country or state where the water or the type of food might influence your reaction to the drug.

One drug listing in the *PDR* reads:

> . . . Before initiating this (medicine) the following procedures are recommended:
> —detailed history and physical examination:
> —this therapy should be prescribed after a critical benefit-to-risk appraisal in patients with history of cardiac, or renal damage, history of adverse hematological reaction to other drugs, or who have had interrupted courses of therapy with "X" (drug name);
> —complete pretreatment blood counts, including platelet and possibly reticulocyte and serum iron should be obtained. Any significant abnormalities should rule out use. . .
> —these same tests should be repeated at frequent intervals, possibly weekly, during the first three months of therapy.

The warning goes on the advise that the possible adverse reactions could include dizziness, drowsiness, nausea, vomiting, aplastic anemia, jaundice, and hepatitis.

If your doctor has never discussed with you the possible consequences of the drug being ordered, ask the necessary questions to elicit this information. Ask about possible tests the manufacturer recommends doing before assigning the medication; ask what the side-effects are likely to be; ask if this is considered a normal dose, or is it larger or smaller than is usually given?

If you don't get complete answers, check for yourself that the medication ordered doesn't require some specific or particular kind of testing to be done *before taking it*. Neglecting this could be harmful to your health.

Tell the doctor that you want to be monitored carefully while taking the medication to make sure serious side-effects do not develop. Find out whether the possible side effects of this medication will mean that you might become drowsy and that driving would be dangerous, that your vision might become blurred, or that you might not be able to eat certain foods. Drugs are, after all, chemical substances foreign to the body, and all have side effects of some kind. The side effects might be internal and not readily apparent. If a side effect does develop, make sure you can get hold of your doctor immediately and stop taking the medication.

Check that the medications you are taking on a regular basis, such as vitamins or antacids, will not block the drugs you are being ordered to take, or make the medication more virulent. Discuss this with your doctor.

Make sure you understand whether the medication ordered for you is to relieve pain or an uncomfortable condition, or whether it is intended to help cure the disease. Tranquilizing someone so that the illness does not seem so stressful does not effect a cure. Be sure to check.

Some experienced clinicians believe that fewer than two dozen drugs are all that would be required to treat 99 percent of the conditions people go to doctors for; others believe that up to four dozen would treat 98 percent. In any event, the oversupply of names, titles, and claims held out for new and wonderful cure-alls are not always true, and past claims for glorious breakthroughs are today often a source of embarrassment.[8]

Medicine and its drugs cannot cure the process of aging and its consequent disabilities, yet this is the area of greatest prescription overload. Medicine can do very little with cardiovascular diseases, most cancers, arthritis, or even the common cold.

Progress in medicine rarely has been made through huge research efforts, or even by doctors. More often, it has been ushered in by "eager beavers" working in individual laboratories in their own homes or offices. Nurse Kenny in Australia found it necessary to set up little hospitals of her own to train other nurses in her techniques of treating infantile paralysis victims before she was taken seriously by doctors. Two scientists, Frederick Banting and Charles Best, discovered insulin while working in the attic of their home.[9] Physicist Dr. Allan McLeod Cormack and his friend, an electronics engineer, Godfrey N. Hounsfield, et al., evolved the CAT-scanner (Computerized Axial Tomography Scanner) that can do a 360° picture of small areas of the body.[10]

The flood of new drugs in the beginning of the twentieth century was not closely examined until the United States Food and Drug Administration turned its attention to the 4,300 prescription drugs that had appeared on the market between the end of the Second World War and 1962. The FDA found that only two out of every five drugs tested were effective, and many on the market were considered dangerous. Among the drugs that met the FDA standards, few were any better than what they had been created to replace.[11]

Diagnostic and therapeutic interventions that really do more good than harm are extremely inexpensive. Most are designed and packaged for self-use or self-application by any adult.

Doctors and those dedicated to the medical viewpoint argue that sick people are nervous and worried and are not competent to handle the job of self-treatment. They point out that when a member of a doctor's own family is ill, another physician is called. What they do not mention is that many effective medications being offered today are oldtime recipes or rediscovered herbs and remedies. In the past, most of these items were either in the home medicine chest or available from a nearby householder who made them up as required.

Some drugs are ordered as "delaying actions." The person who wakes in the night with an excruciatingly painful headache because of blocked sinuses is a typical example. The "take two aspirins and call me in the morning" ploy was probably originated for these long-suffering people. Aspirins effectively numb the aching areas and let you go back to sleep. In the morning the headache may be a memory, and the entire incident considered too unimportant to demand rigorous attention—by your doctor.

The condition is a common one and the suffering is great. Why not, then, do something that would remove the infection in the sinus cavities so that there would be no recurrence of the blinding headaches, the stuffed-up nose, the teary eyes—and the lost work time? Half-measures in the treatment of sinus conditions have been pervasive. Upon investigation it is discovered that the cure is cheap and simple, ruling out interest by the pharmaceutical companies.

Try this: At the local drugstore, buy an all-glass nasal douche. Do not use a forced douche with a bulb, as the high pressure can force the infection further into the head. Clean and sterilize it. Then you need only a drinking glass, the nasal douche, some hot water and a small amount of table salt for the treatment. Fill the drinking glass half full of water, as hot as you can comfortably stand on the inside of your nose. Add a pinch of salt and stir. Fill the nasal douche with the mixture and prepare to attack the problem. Stand near the sink and put your head back—way, way back. Then put the pointed end into the nasal passage while you keep your finger on the little raised tube-like projection. When your head is far back, raise your finger and let the hot water into the nose. The water will go back and into the throat, and come out the mouth, clearing the obstruction before it. Let the water drop back as far as possible, a little at a time. When you have cleared one side, do the other if you have a problem with that too.

If you have had sinus troubles for a considerable period of time, you will need daily treatments for a little while before you can control the condition.

The alternative is to find a doctor who is sympathetic to this simple remedy. First, ask your doctor to determine if you will have any allergic reaction to this method. If you are not allergic, have the doctor prescribe a tiny bit of an antibiotic, to which you are not sensitive, in some distilled water. Use this in place of the salt-and-water combination. It is more expensive and might be slightly faster, but either one will do the trick.

The whole problem of drugs is in need of review, according to Dr. Illich. All drugs have side-effects for someone, whether sold by prescription or over-the-counter. The doctor who tells you that a drug has no side-effects is placating you, soothing you into acceptance—at a risk.

NOTES

1. Ivan Illich, *Medical Nemesis*, p. 70.
2. Ibid., p. 71.
3. Ibid., p. 73.
4. Mark Dowie et al., "The Illusion of Safety," *Mother Jones Magazine*, Vol. 7 No. 5, p. 47.
5. Ibid., pp. 36–49.
6. Ibid., p. 48.
7. James Dunlap, *Medical Negligence*, p. 12.
8. Ivan Illich, *Medical Nemesis*, p. 74.
9. James Wasco, *Not For Doctors Only*, p. 86.
10. Ibid., p. 108.
11. Cathey Pinckney and Edward R. Pinckney, *The Patient's Guide to Medical Tests*, p. xiv.

8

The Public Library
as a Health Resource

A month has passed. You may have been back to the doctor at least once, and the medication you did not seem to tolerate well or that was not having any effect on your condition may have been changed. What do you do next?

Why not do some research on your own? Through research you may determine whether you are being diagnosed properly and whether the medication being offered is appropriate for the condition or symptoms experienced.

Few people are aware of the amount of medical information available in their local public library. Almost all public libraries, even the branches, have at least one medical dictionary. It might not be the latest edition, but at least it will give you some clue regarding your doctor's diagnosis.

In the card catalog SUBJECT section, look under the headings of "DICTIONARIES, MEDICAL" or "MEDICAL DICTIONARIES."

If you are unfamiliar with the card catalog, ask your librarian for assistance. When you find the card, there will be notations on it. The numbers on the upper left-hand side of the card, using the Dewey decimal system, are important. They will help you locate not only the particular book you want, but also most of the medical data in that particular library. All the strictly medical books will be in the same general area.

If the medical dictionary is not on the shelf, it may be available through the reference librarian. Excellent dictionaries include: *Taber's Cyclopedic Medical Dictionary*, edited by Clayton L. Thomas and published by F. A. Davis Company; or *Melloni's Illustrated Medical Dictionary* by Ida Dox, John Melloni Biagio and Gilbert Eisner, published by Williams and Wilkins; or *Dorland's Illustrated Medical Dictionary*, published by Saunders and Company.

If the medical dictionary is not a recent one, ask that a newer one be borrowed from another library. The librarian will give you the necessary forms to fill out so the book may be borrowed for your use. You will be notified when it comes in.

With the notes you made to take to the doctor's office, plus the ones you took at the time of your visit, open the medical dictionary to the alphabetical index at the back. Find the diagnosis the doctor gave you. Use the photocopying machine in the library or copy down by hand *everything* that appears under this heading. Then add the following important information, called the bibliography:

—The name of the author or editor as it appears on the title page of the book, last name first. If the names given are editors rather than authors, make note of that too.

—The title of the book in its entirety, just as it appears on the title page, include any subtitle given. If there is a similarity to another title, the subtitle information will help to clarify which book you have been using.

—Turn the title page over and find the date of the copyright, which will follow a little "c" inside a circle. If the name and address of the publisher do not appear on the title page, you will find them on the reverse side of the title page.

This bibliographic information (referred to by librarians as "the biblio") should be added to any copies or duplicated material you collect in the field of medicine. It will help to establish the authenticity of the data, if necessary, at some later date.

Note the date of the copyright before you copy anything. There have been so many advances in medicine in the last few years that it is necessary, in doing intelligent up-to-date research, to consult dictionaries and medical books published fairly recently. An over-simplified explanation is nearly useless, and one that has not taken into account the new and advanced methods of discovery and treatment will not help you much either.

All medical dictionaries have several things in common: they will explain how to pronounce the name of the disease, will give a run-down of the forms of the disease, and will list some of the symptoms. If the words in the explanations are complicated, look these up too. The more fluently you can use a medical term, the more seriously medical people will treat your questions and challenges. Often there are sketches or pictures illustrating the text: some even in color.

Let's try one together. The problem of loss of hair has ceased to be only a male preserve. Women, for many reasons rarely researched, have been having problems with baldness, and there is a good deal more of it than is being recognized. Let's do some research on this subject.

Using *Taber's Cyclopedic Medical Dictionary*, look up "hair." You will find a clear description as well as a color picture of hair structures. If you read the text, you will find the sentence:

> ". . . Baldness or alopecia results when replacements fail to keep
> up with hair loss . . ."

In this instance, the text indicates that the word "alopecia" means baldness. Clearly if you look up "baldness," you will find: *See:* alopecia.

Under alopecia you will find, in parentheses, the correct pronunciation. The derivation is given next, and the definition follows.

"Etiol." stands for etiology and is the probable cause for the disease.

Treatment is discussed in understandable terms. The forms of alopecia are listed in alphabetical order. The small "a" before the fourteen listings stands for "alopecia" and entries should be read: "alopecia adnata," "alopecia areata," and on down the list. Some of the descriptive terms are understandable, neurotica being closely related to the word neurotic, that we see so often in magazines and newspapers, and the explanation confirms this: loss of hair following a nervous disease or injury to the nervous system.

If a definition of the information your doctor gave you is sufficient for your needs, your research is over.

However, if you want the alternative diagnoses for the condition you are researching, you will need to go onto the next step: the use of a manual or reference book. If the library you are using is large and well-stocked with medical data, it may have a book that discusses precisely the condition you are researching. Many medical books are devoted entirely to a single diagnosis or condition. If the library does not own a book that serves your purpose, ask that one be borrowed through Interlibrary Loan.

The reference librarian who usually takes care of the interlibrary loans in the public library will give you a slip to fill out, and the book will be sent from a cooperating library to your local library for your use. This should take a week or two.

You might start with requesting any of the following excellent, but by no means only, reference books available:

—Berkow, Robert, et al., editor. *The Merck Manual of Diagnosis and Therapy*. Merck, Sharp and Dohme Research Laboratories.
—Harrison, Tinsley Randolph. *Harrison's Principles of Internal Medicine*. McGraw-Hill. (This title may come in two volumes.)
—Conn and Conn, editors. *Current Diagnosis*. Saunders Publishing Company.

Manuals are published to update the knowledge of doctors in their specific fields. These are offered in the various specialties and will provide a picture of the various forms an illness might take within that particular part of the body.

If the manual you have used does not give sufficient information about the conditions of interest to you, there are other books to which you may refer. To find them, turn to *Books in Print*, published by R. R. Bowker.

Books in Print (BIP) is published every year in three volumes: the author guide, the title guide, and the subject guide. The subject guide is the one you will want to use at this time. You may find what you are looking for under Medical Care, Medical Centers, Medical Fees, etc. The section on medical subjects is quite extensive, but do not overlook the possibility of finding a book whose title might interest you under the diagnosis itself. For instance, alopecia is not listed as one of the subjects in the subject guide, but diabetes is. Make note of the fact too that psychiatry and psychology are not listed in the medical section at all, but are listed separately under "P."

Books in Print is usually available at the desk of the reference librarian or may be consulted at any book store. (Bowker also publishes *BIP* in paperback.) The books listed in *BIP* are available for purchase during the year shown on the spine. The book you are looking for could have been published a year or two earlier. Older books are listed if they are still being published and distributed. You may need to use the *Cumulative Book Index (CBI)* to locate books on your topic which are no longer being published. *CBI* lists all books published in English.

If you locate a book of interest to you by a specific author, you may find the author has published additional books on the same or similar subject. In that case, refer to the author guide and examine the titles of the other books that author has written. You might find one that interests you.

If the book you want is an inexpensive paperback, Interlibrary Loan may not be able to get it for you. The life of a paperback is not very long, so libraries prefer to keep them for use of their own clientele.

Copy down *all* the information in *BIP* regarding the book you want. Make careful note of the author, the exact title, plus the copyright date and the publisher. The bibliography is *BIP.* Note the volume number, the year, and the page number. If you find you need to check again and return to this page, you will have simplified the process considerably.

Under the heading of "Medical" there will also be a short list of the other subject titles that *BIP* would suggest you use to find other listings.

If you have not found something that interests you, or the listings seem formidable in length, you may consult *Medical Books in Print.* Sometimes this is difficult to find in a public library. This book lists all the medical books available for purchase in the year shown on the spine. Make sure that the manual or reference book you are requesting has been published fairly recently before you take the time and trouble to use it for research. Check this before you start.

The best way to approach research in a manual or reference book is to work from the index at the back of the book. Find the diagnosis you are interested in, listed in alphabetical order. Turn to the page or pages listed and concentrate on what seems pertinent to your search. Copy down everything that appears on the subject, and do not forget to note the bibliography. Using the copy machine makes this job simple; do not forget to add the biblio onto the photocopied sheet before returning the book.

At the end of each short chapter in most manuals or reference books, you may find a list of books and articles that delve further into the subject. These might be useful to you because the author of the item you are copying has used them for preparing the paper. The biblio here is the article itself, the title of the book, the author or editor, the city and publisher, and the page number.

The notebook you are organizing of material from the library and the doctor's office should be presenting a series of words, phrases and diagnoses to which you can refer as you proceed with your research.

9

Using the Medical Library

A week or ten days—maybe even two weeks—have passed and the librarian at the local library informs you that the books you want to see are "on reserve" and therefore not available for Interlibrary Loan. What do you do?

If you have not already done so, now is the time to plan to visit the nearest hospital medical library. Before going, however, be aware of some important considerations about using medical libraries in hospitals.

—*Telephone for an appointment* so that you will not be using the books, audio-visual materials, and vertical files during their heaviest use time. When interns, doctors, nurses, and social workers are there in full force, they have priority, and rightly so.

Telephoning will give the medical librarian an opportunity to plan for your visit and to make sure that it does not conflict with other appointments or the needs of the primary users of the library.

—Make sure you give yourself enough time to learn your way around the library, where to find things, and whom to ask for what.

—Leave children at home. They can be a distraction to you and others.

—Take your own paper, pencils, pens, and erasers with you. Be prepared to take the notes you will need without bothering other people.

—Make sure you have plenty of change. You will need nickels and dimes to use the copy machine. After the first visit you'll know where the machine is and what coins it takes.

—*Do as much as you can for yourself.* This is one of the most important suggestions for the use of the medical library. The less bother you are during the time you are there, the less objection anyone will make to your being there, even during busy periods.

The medical library will probably arrange its books according to the classification system originated by the National Library of Medicine (NLM) which is very different from the Dewey decimal system found in public libraries. However, it will not be difficult for you to find what you are looking for because the shelves should be labeled and the books will follow a line of progress. In the NLM system, most of the medical books you will be using will have a code that starts with a "W." It will then go to "WA," "WB," "WC," and so forth, all the way to "WZ."

Each of the lettered categories represents a separate medical discipline. For instance, titles shelved under "WS" discuss children, and "WZ" is concerned with the history of medicine. A complete outline of the subject classification system should be posted in the medical library to assist the staff as well as visitors.

Before starting, consider the nature of books themselves. The character of a book indicates if the material it contains is not brand new. Presumably it could take five years or more to collect the information for a book in the field of medicine. Scientific professions require that the discussions and statistics they accept be proved over and over again. It takes time to write and organize the material into understandable and usable form and to find a publisher. More time elapses before the book is published and placed on the medical library bookshelves for use. Because we have grown accustomed to instant reporting in the media, the time lag of medical book publishing is difficult to understand and accept. The material you will find in these books, however, is the basis upon which your own physician assesses symptoms. Do not hesitate to use what is offered in these texts with the proviso that the books are fairly recent.

NOTE: If the librarian objects to your use of the medical library, remind him/her that the library is obliged to be available to the public on a reasonable basis. The hospital receives a tax exemption because it provides a public service, and therefore it does not pay any taxes toward fire, water, police, street cleaning, or any other services received from the city, state, or federal government—to which you are a heavy and regular contributor!

Don't take no for an answer!

The books you need on almost every subject in the field of medicine should be there. Just as in the public library, the card file is available. It is usually divided into two sections, the first a listing of author and title of books, and the second, the subject file.

If you already have the titles or authors of books you want to see, you're all set. Note the number shown on the left hand side of the catalog card on your notepaper, and then hunt through the shelves for the book you want.

I would suggest that two lists be kept in the back of your notebook; the first will list the books you would like to see, with all the information to help you locate them. The second, on a separate page, will list the books you have found and consulted. Not only should all the bibliographic information about each of these be written down, but also a two- or three-line summary of what the book contains should be noted, so it will not be necessary to hunt for it again in the future. Copy down the numbers that will help find the books on the shelves, and you will not have to look them up a second time.

Almost all medical libraries have the same classification system. One of the advantages for you is that the number, taken down from the card file in this library, will probably locate the book for you under the same number in the next medical library you use.

In the manual or reference books you will be able to collect information not available from the dictionary. There will probably be an expanded list of symptoms, a prognosis (the potential for recovery) as well as suggested treatments.

Now turn in the index to your symptoms. Copy out the suggestions for further research given under each of these headings.

For instance, in Conn's *Current Therapy,* you will find: *allergic reactions,* and a list that includes "lips," "drugs," "insect stings," "insulin," "phenytoin" (a drug of choice for epilepsy), and "transfusion." Each of these suggests another area of research and the possibility that a variety of conditions may be giving the allergic reactions. Turning to each of the suggested pages will give an explanation which may sound complicated until you read it over carefully a few times.

Group your notes as you proceed. If you come across several diagnoses in your research, perhaps the best way to work on more than one diagnosis at a time is to head up one sheet for each diagnosis, adding symptoms as you go. When you have finished noting your own symptoms and the diagnoses you have collected, you must decide whether any subject is worth investigating further.

In looking up symptoms in the reference books, try to use as specific a symptom as you can. Generalized symptoms such as "headache" or "nausea" will produce such long lists of possible diagnoses that you might not be able to concentrate on anything that would be helpful. While you are being as specific as possible, do not overlook the possibility that more than one disease or condition may be present and need to be researched.

Guide yourself in your research by using the same clues that your doctor would use, such as your own past illnesses and the illnesses of your family. The amount of pain an individual can bear is peculiar to that individual, and people differ remarkably in the amount of pain they can stand. Therefore, "pain," in itself, is not a good symptom for research unless the site and distribution of the pain is taken into account. Establish whether the pain is constant. Does pain occur at night, during the day, after eating, during certain times of the month? Keep these questions in mind as you go through the literature.

If the book you are using does not offer the information you had hoped to find, do not hesitate to ask the medical librarian to suggest another. One note about the role of the librarian. It is illegal for medical librarians to even suggest a diagnosis. People who did so would be guilty of "practicing medicine without a license" even if they have the same disease and recognize the symptoms. Medical librarians cannot help you with a diagnosis even if they want to. They dare not. But they can suggest other books for you to use to find the information you are seeking.

If your work was carefully organized and collected, the data you set out to compile are becoming clearer. You now have a principal diagnosis offered by your physician, a list of symptoms, plus other diagnoses found in the text of the manuals and reference books you have consulted. For many people, a cursory research session of books available will not suffice. If you wish to uncover the most recent writings on the newest therapies, you will need to consult a variety of medical journals. The techniques of researching journals are not difficult to learn. The library will have a list of the journals to which it subscribes; if the list cannot be found near the card file, the librarian may have it. The most comprehensive journal in any medical library is *Index Medicus (IM)*. This large paperbound volume is issued monthly by the National Library of Medicine. The first one of the year, issued in January, comes out in two volumes; all the other issues are only one volume. These are the most up-to-date of the listings that you are going to use. The information represents the medical information gathered from thousands of medical journals all over the world, in all languages. Each of the paperbound issues is divided into two portions, the first is a listing of articles according to subject. The second portion is an alphabetical listing of the authors of the articles, plus the titles of the articles and other pertinent material. If you are researching a subject, it is not likely you will use the second portion of *IM*, but don't rule it out.

To use *IM*, start with the diagnosis your doctor gave you. If it is a fairly large subject like diabetes or kidney disease, for instance, you will find the main listing subdivided in alphabetical order, according to the various forms of the disease. In bold type under the main heading you will find suggestions of other related subjects you might research. At first glance there does not seem to be any order to the listings, but you will note they are in alphabetical order according to the names of the journals in which they appear. The title of a journal called *Abstracts for Social Workers,* for instance, would come first, if there was an article in it under this heading. An article in the journal *Headache* or *Journal of the American Medical Association* would come under "H" or "J" respectively.

Articles in foreign languages often are not translated anywhere in their entirety. However, there may be a short synopsis in English at the very beginning of the article. This will be noted in *IM*. If the title of the article appears in brackets, the article is in a foreign language. Which foreign language it appears in is noted at the lower right-hand corner of the call-out, abbreviated but clearly indicated. Do not call for that article unless you can read that language fluently. A medical translator can take on the job for you, but this would be rather expensive.

The articles themselves are likely to be written by a doctor, social worker, nurse or psychologist about something new or unusual. These professionals write to indicate their interest in problems other readers of these journals might be researching. It is a way for them to say to the rest of their profession: "I would like to hear from someone interested in the same type of work, therapy or ideas...." In some cases the author would like to hear from someone willing to share the results.

Many, but not all, journals in a medical library specialize in only one field of medicine. One journal is called *Headache,* another *Heart,* and others are devoted exclusively to urology, psychoanalysis, retardation, and other specialties. Only a few journals will be of interest to you.

Look over the titles of the articles carefully. Unlike fiction or political books, medical titles almost always reveal exactly the subject being discussed.

Another resource is *Cumulative Index Medicus (CIM).* These books are a bound cumulation of *IM*s. They represent a whole year of medical articles grouped under their proper subject and author headings. Each subject in *CIM* represents all that was written on that particular subject for that entire year, including data from foreign journals. The year covered is noted on the spine of the volume, and like any encyclopedia, the letters it covers are noted too. The subject section of the entire year's collection might include as many as six or more volumes, depending upon the number of listings that year.

Do not become discouraged by the long lists of items in *CIM.* To speed up the search, you might choose only articles in English or discard any subject heading that may not seem pertinent.

Note too that the National Library of Medicine puts out its own listings of literature on particular subjects. You might be lucky enough to find that they have issued such a list recently in a field that interests you. The listings for these, free of charge to the medical library, are on the inside front cover of *IM.* If these are requested by the medical librarian it may take up to a month to get them from NLM.

The listings in *IM* and *CIM* (called "call-outs" by librarians) pack much information into a small space. Elements of the listings are as follows:

—the title of the article, followed by a period. If there is a colon or a semi-colon, it is usual to add a qualifier or a subtitle to the title;

—the name of the author. The last name will be given first, the first name next, and lastly the initial or middle name. Sometimes there will be just a last name and an initial, especially where the name is unusual and not likely to be confused with other contributors who write on the same or similar subjects;

—the name of the journal printed in bold face. Sometimes this is an abbreviation. Consult the front of the *IM,* where you will find a listing of the journals "covered" by *IM,* or ask the medical librarian;

—a series of numbers and letters after the name of the journal which must be copied down correctly if you want to find the article. The first number is the year the article was published; next is the monthly issue the article is in; then the volume number; then the issue number and after the colon, the pages on which you can find the article. The page numbers will give some clue about the length of the article. Remember there is advertising in medical journals, and the page listings do not always reflect the number of pages given over to a discussion of the subject.

Once in a while there will be an additional piece of information for the researcher such as: (70 ref.). This means that at the end of that particular article, there are seventy listings of other articles the authors have examined while preparing to write the article. However, a word of warning here: frequently doctors and nurses feel their prestige would suffer if there were too few listings at the end of their article. Sometimes the listings note articles to which the author never referred.

A typical heading might be "Diabetes, prevention and control." The reference would read:

Prevention and treatment of diabetic complications. Levin, M. E. et al. **Arch Intern Med** 1980 May: 140(5) 691–6

The title of the article is "Prevention and Treatment of Diabetic Complications," the author is M. E. Levin and others (et al.), the article appears in *Archives of Internal Medicine* for 1980, in the May issue, volume 140, Issue 5. The article appears on pages 691 through 696.

Because the May issue was number 5, the journal probably comes out once a month, with the first volume being January and the last for the year being December. Note the fact that some of the journals have a fiscal year beginning in May, June, or July. In this case, the fifth volume would be a month other than May. Sometimes only four, six or nine issues are published each year. That is why every piece of the information is important to your finding the article you want.

Scanning a whole year's listings under each heading may take some time, but it will be worth your while. At the end of the search, you should have a fairly good idea of whether the information you want is going to be available under that particular subject heading.

Don't forget also to check listings in the *CIM* of last year, the year before, and even recent previous years. Much medical information is overlooked by doctors and other professionals until some time after its introduction. Papers may have to be presented at medical conventions and in journals several times before interest is aroused sufficiently to interest others in doing further research in the field.

The medical librarian will have the request forms you will have to fill out to obtain the articles. If you fill in all the spaces, you will have given the information you found listed in *IM* or *CIM*. Remember to take down the biblio! In this instance, the biblio is the year, the volume, the issue, and the page number of the *IM* or the *CIM* you used for this reference.

You will probably be asked for the following information on the request form. Be sure it is filled out completely, so that the librarian can help you find what you want with as little trouble as possible.

1. Date of request
2. Indicate whether the item you want is a journal article, a book, or audio-visual material.
3. The author of the article, last name first
4. Title of the item
5. The biblio
6. Your name and where you can be reached by telephone when the material is reproduced for you
7. Note the last date this information would be useful to you, so that a "hurry-call" can be put on it if it is an emergency.

After you have written up a separate ticket for each article you want, check with the list of journals available in that particular medical library. You might make a small pencil mark on the upper right- or left-hand corner of the ticket if the library does not subscribe to that particular journal. Put these tickets away for now. They will be discussed later.

The remaining tickets refer to journal articles available in the medical library you are now in. At first you might need some help locating the journals, but after that you will find it simple to go right to the item. Examine each article before you take it to the copying machine. If it is not interesting to you, you will be saving time, money, and effort by rejecting it at this point.

If the information on your subject is sparse and you want to spend the time and effort to research the foreign language call-outs, you might refer to the Translation Registry Index to see if the papers have been translated. By good fortune, you might find that someone else was anxious for information in that field, and had the foreign-language article translated. Ask the librarian to check with other libraries to locate a copy of the Translation Registry booklets.

Working carefully and methodically through *IM* and *CIM*, you still might not find the information you need. In this case you might try looking up the symptoms instead of the diagnosis.

When you have located the article in the journal, you will note right under the title there is a short synopsis of the article. If the article seems to have the information you want, make a copy of it. Scan the list of papers and books the author mentions at the end of the article, and follow up on any that might interest you.

You may also refer to the "Vertical File." This is the librarian's term for a file used to collect articles returned by patrons who have requested material unavailable in this library. Use the same subject headings in searching through the vertical file as you used in *IM* or *CIM*. The folders should be organized along the same subject lines. Over a period of time some interesting and relevant articles should have been collected. In some libraries, the articles taken from the vertical file may be borrowed or kept without charge. Although the material was probably not collected within the last year or two, it still might be the latest reporting on that subject.

Aside from cooperating libraries, the federal government, armed forces, and health departments on state and federal levels might have data of interest. Some information is available for purchase, but this is inclined to be expensive, so a central cooperating group often purchases and shares the use of these items.

Another area of research open to the public in the small or medium-sized local medical library is the audio-visual department. The kind of equipment the hospital has been able to afford limits the ways in which it can provide information to its staff and to the public. A listing of audio-visuals owned by other cooperating libraries should be available; arranging for their use with the medical librarian will not delay your research for long. You might be lucky enough to find something to view on an audio or video cassette in the field you are researching.

Slides, moving pictures, video-tapes, discs and cassettes for tape recorders are available in the medical field. Combinations of any two or three of these might prove as useful and interesting as any journal article. You can always turn the machine back to the beginning to view the whole program over again. It is now standard practice in many teaching hospitals to have closed-circuit television in operating rooms and lecture halls, so the audio-visuals available may be quite sophisticated. You may need to make an appointment to view the audio-visual materials.

The local public library often has cassettes, video-cassettes or film projectors that you may borrow. If the library cannot make these available, a local supplier who works with public schools might allow you to rent or borrow a piece of equipment. Be sure the wiring in your house is compatible with the wiring of the machinery you are borrowing or renting. Don't guess. Have someone trained in the field check this matter for you. Usually a booklet will accompany the machine giving comprehensive instructions in the care and operation of the machinery to help prevent costly accidents.

Note that many of the audio-visuals distributed to hospitals are made by pharmaceutical companies. In many cases, they are aimed at interns training to be doctors and "pin-stripers" training to be nurses. These audio-visuals are, in a sense, marketing devices which suggest that medication is the most effective avenue for treatment. Give your attention to the basic discussion of the possible etiology (cause) of the disease or the operation taking place. Films, film-strips and slides with Spanish voice-over are also available.

There are audio-visual programs aimed directly at non-physicians such as nurses, dental students, hospital kitchen workers and many others. While most of these are concerned with teaching medical information to professionals, the words used are more understandable and less technical. Try them and see if they are suitable for your purpose.

Browse through the medical library and see if there are other areas of use to you. Ask questions about anything of interest. The librarian will be delighted with your interest, and you will have a better understanding of how the medical library can contribute to your knowledge.

10

Visiting a Larger
Medical Library

Turn your attention to the slips of paper you've accumulated representing articles that are not in the local medical library you have been using. There are several ways of dealing with these tickets.

Most large hospital libraries have books which list the journals available in other medical libraries in the state. You may be charged for obtaining articles from these cooperating institutions, although it is common for in-house staff to receive this service free of charge. Ask the medical librarian what the charge would be for sending articles from these other medical libraries before you make a formal request. Then you will have to decide whether the expense is worth it to you.

If the expense is too great, or if it seems to involve too much investment over a period of time, ask to study the listings. Note which hospital(s) have the largest number of the journals you want to see. Then, if at all possible, plan to visit the one with the largest and most complete collection.

There is a tremendous advantage in being able to go where there is large journal coverage. You may do your own copying at a minimum cost, and you will usually find a larger collection of dictionaries, manuals, and audio-visuals for looking up the "pure medicalese" as well as the more obscure medical data found in the discussions of the articles.

The same procedures you used in your local medical library will be useful in a larger one. Most likely, this library will be using the National Library of Medicine classification system, so you may refer back to the numbers and titles of the books you found originally.

Where two medical institutions are fairly close to each other, they may cooperate and supplement each other's journal collection because the budget crunch has affected them too. This means that you might visit a second large institution to complete the research you started nearby.

If you still have not located material which really answers your questions, there is another option. Some medical libraries at larger hospitals have computers for research purposes. Give your list of terms and the original diagnosis to the medical librarian and ask that these be fed into the computer. Be sure to ask what this will cost first!

If the computer terminal is not housed in this library, the librarian may have access to one through another library's "little black box." The librarian may telephone the other library to give them the data. The main frame of the computer is at the National Library of Medicine, and a printout will be transmitted to your terminal.

Medical journals are carefully examined for additional subject indexing for the computer. In *IM* or *CIM* they might be listed only under one or two headings. The same article may turn up under several other important headings in the computer listing. You have a much better chance of finding the subject you are concerned with, if it exists, through the use of the computer. The printout should not take long, but the price is sometimes greater than you had expected.

Using a distant medical library does have its drawbacks, so plan well before you go. The books are not available for loan to you unless you have a friend in the institution who will let you borrow them in his/ her name.

If you must check the material you have extracted again, or have forgotton to note a page number or the spelling of the author's name, the trip may be too long for such a chore to be redone. In the case of the author's name, don't forget to try using *IM* or *CIM*, which deal with authors' names, if you have the exact title of the article itself. It can be looked up in the second half of the *IM* or *CIM*, which will list both the author's name and the title of the journal article. If it is a book, however, you will find the listing in *Books in Print* or *Medical Books in Print,* both of which are probably available in the medical library.

If you haven't written the title clearly enough to read and list it properly, look it up under the author's name, but the correct spelling must be used. In looking up the title, remember that words like "the," "a" and "an" are not used in alphabetizing a title, and names starting with "Mc" or "Mac" are treated the same, under "Mac" at the beginning of the M's.

There should be a correspondingly larger collection of audio-visuals as well as data in the pamphlet file in the larger institution. If you are lucky, this may be a teaching institution, in which case you might find that interesting audio-visuals are charged out and are being used in another department. This means that the materials are current and up-to-date. Do not hesitate either to wait for them to be free or to make an appointment to view them at a later date.

You may be able to have audio-visuals, tapes or films loaned to your hospital medical library, where you may see them at your convenience. There is often a backlog of cataloging to be done in every library, especially with audio-visuals, so the material you find available during your visit to the larger hospital may not have been added yet to the lists sent around the state. In that case you would not have learned this information was available unless you visited this larger hospital library!

Clear ahead of time with the medical librarian of your local hospital your use of the larger medical facility. A letter that will earn you the privilege of borrowing a book or a pamphlet may be given to you. Ask at that time, too, if there is a pick-up service that serves your "home" medical library. You might find that the materials you borrow may be picked up at the "home" medical library and returned for you. That would save a trip or having to send them by mail, and would get them there faster as well.

If you must send materials back by mail, make sure they arrive in the same good condition in which you received them. Special insulated envelopes are available for sending delicate materials through the mail. *Do not fail to do this,* or your borrowing privileges might be curtailed. When the time comes to ask again, you will find the library very firm indeed about turning you down!

If you have decided to have a computer printout done, the medical librarian will help you to choose the two or three key words that will bring titles, authors, and journal names to you. Consider taking along two or three large-size mailing envelopes, stamped, self-addressed, and ready to go. If these are left with the librarian, the printout will be sent to you.

In general, medical librarians are helpful and knowledgeable in their field. Give them an understanding of what you are searching for, some warning that you are coming so that someone can plan to spend some time alone with you, and enough time to get the information together for you. Remember, the librarian's own work must come first, especially during an emergency.

You have now completed the round of what Western medicine has to offer in written and audio-visual materials. The data you have gathered should cover what your doctor or consultant would have to offer as a solution to your problem. Does it?

11

Alternative Forms
of Therapy

What do you do when you have exhausted your patience, your pocketbook and your time trying to get medical solutions that elude you?

There are other forms of therapy, most of them not recognized by our standard medical profession but used successfully in other parts of the world.

The National Women's Health Network, for instance, is trying to respond to the growing number of people who have been given inappropriate or hazardous medical care. This includes contraceptive injuries, diagnostic errors and treatments, surgery done unnecessarily or badly, drug therapies incorrectly prescribed, unnecessary hysterectomies, birth defects caused by drugs prescribed during pregnancy or trauma during pregnancy, and severe reactions to experimental or unapproved drugs. They can be reached at the National Women's Health Network, 224 Seventh Street S.E., Washington, DC 20003. Consultation with their litigation service is free of charge.

The erosion of the doctor-patient relationship in recent years is pervasive. Doctors, nurses, and pharmaceutical companies must learn that people talk to each other about them—with growing dismay. Eventually, it is hoped that those doctors who provide inadequate care will find it healthier for their pocketbooks and their prestige to raise their standards of service.

Meanwhile, alternative forms of therapy used for centuries in other countries are available to those who have not been helped by conventional Western medicine. One may not find practitioners of these therapies in every community, but good health and a feeling of well-being are worth the effort required to locate them.

The following descriptions of alternative therapies will provide a brief overview of each method. These descriptions will give you a point from which to launch further research if the method appeals to you. One of the advantages of some of these forms of therapy is that they may be carried out to supplement your doctor's care, and a few of them you may do for yourself.

Acupuncture[1]

Practiced by the Chinese for more than five thousand years, acupuncture is used to treat a wide variety of medical problems throughout the Far East, Great Britain, Eastern and Western Europe, the Soviet Union, and the rest of Asia as well. Few licensed medical practitioners in the United States have learned the technique, and it is still considered "experimental" in Western medicine. But estimates are that more people have been treated by acupuncture in the course of history than by all other known systems of medicine combined.

The Chinese philosophy underlying acupuncture treatment is that disease originates from within the individual and has a personal if not a physical cause. In contrast, the philosophy of the Middle Ages, in Europe particularly, considered disease a catastrophe visited upon people for evil deeds they had done, a punishment. Disease was not controllable because it emanated from outside the patient's being.

Chinese beliefs concerning illness divide the causes of disease into two classifications: the first being the outside world of meteorological conditions, in a very broad sense, and the other, the emotions. The Chinese believe that weather, wind, and storms have an effect on people and how they feel. They talk of how a person can be inside a warm room away from a storm and still feel poorly, because of the meterological disturbances outdoors.

The "inner causes," according to this philosophy, might in our terms be called "psychosomatic"—the physical results of uncontrolled emotion. Even a passing emotion may be harmful and may give rise to physical disease. A normally healthy person will recover from illness as soon as the situation that caused the "uncontrolled emotion" alters for the better. If the person is depressed (ill) for a long period of time, treating the offended part of the body will help to clear up the condition—if the patient also makes the effort to help him/herself.

In the Chinese philosophy, food is considered the source of energy in life. The body must extract the essence from foods and distribute it to the rest of the body through the spleen. Excessive food, excessive labor, excessive sexual activity affect particular parts of the body. Moderation in all things is considered the quintessence of existence.

The method of treatment in acupuncture is uncomplicated. Extremely thin gold, silver, or solid stainless steel needles are inserted at various points of the body, left there for a little while, then removed. The practitioner may twirl the needles gently after insertion. In some cases a moss-like substance is wrapped gently around the uppor portion of the needle and set to smouldering.

Some needles are placed far from the site of the injury or the diseased organ, but the reaction time is short—one or two seconds—before some relief is noticeable. Sometimes the placement of the needles seems random, but acupuncturists claim that their therapy readjusts the functions of the internal energy paths related to particular organs. The nerves they touch with the tip of the needles bring relief to sensitive areas and repeated treatment brings the organ into healthy realignment and proper functioning.

After you recover from the first terror of the needles, you will find that the treatment doesn't hurt and doesn't even draw blood. The needles are so fine, often no thicker than a human hair, that you don't really feel them as they are inserted. Their rounded, pencil-tip points push the tissues aside without cutting them. As a result only a slight pinprick is felt when they are inserted, and then a feeling of tingling or a heaviness is experienced. There is no question that acupuncture has provided relief in instances where conventional Western medicine has not.

Some Western physicians shrug off improvement of this nature with the comment that the illness was probably psychosomatic, but in the case of neurological problems it is worth a try. No method in Western medicine does the job adequately. In the case of neuralgia, for instance, the best your doctor can do is inject alcohol at the sight of the pain—in essence, making the nerve drunk until the worst of the pain or irritation passes. Or the doctor may provide a tranquilizer. For extreme pain, some doctors even recommend cutting the nerve itself so that there is no opportunity for healing.

Acupuncture is *not* a cure-all but it is worth investigating. It does seem to affect favorably some areas that Western medicine has not been able to help.

A volunteer in my medical library told me that her daughter, born deaf, was able to hear with a hearing aid when she started kindergarten as long as she had acupuncture on a regular basis. When the acupuncture stopped, the child's ability to hear ceased and they had to start again so she could make a normal adjustment to her peer group.

Many years ago, I traveled to Hong Kong where friends made it possible for me to have treatment for very painful facial neuralgia. When I returned, the doctors I worked with were amused at my claims of relief. Because all of my life I have hovered near the level of anemia, I refused the drug they had offered me. Now, ten years later, I have sensitivity in that same area, but I will still refuse their "medicine" and wait until the pain grows greater to justify another trip to Hong Kong.

Acupuncture in China as well as other parts of the world is used for anesthesia in dental and surgical procedures, for treatment of chronic pain, diseases of deafness, and paralysis. More than 400,000 operations had been performed in China by 1970, since the time the new regime had permitted re-introduction of this ancient technique. About 30 percent of all surgery there is done in this manner.

The results do not seem to be effective with children in many cases, but there are distinct advantages in its use. You are conscious, don't experience nausea and do not have other unpleasant after-effects of anesthetics. You recover more quickly, and rarely experience complications such as pneumonia.

Acupuncture doesn't seem to work with all people, however. If the operation is a long one, the effects of the needles seem to wear off and an alternate form of anesthesia must be used.

Despite wide discussion of acupuncture in newspapers and television programs a few years ago, there has not been any extensive use of acupuncture in medical treatment in this country.

The effect of the treatment is not a steady uphill climb from chronic pain or illness, but a little improvement each time, lasting longer with each treatment. Finally, the effects last long enough to discontinue treatment, temporarily or permanently. Sometimes a setback will occur during the treatment that will affect the placement of the needles for later treatments. The acupuncturist contends it is rare indeed that a person comes for treatment with just one complaint. In addition to the chief complaint, there are usually a number of small, chronic complaints that do not disable but just keep the patient from feeling really well. A small list of the diseases that acupuncture claims to treat with good results are neuralgia, headache, tics, cerebral arteriosclerosis in its early stage, muscular rheumatism, sciatica, cold hands and feet and early rheumatoid or osteoarthritis.

All methods of treatment of diseases give some good results. Without doubt, the patient's anticipation of improvement or recovery has much to do with the good progress of an illness. The bright expectations of the therapist also may make a valuable contribution to the prognosis and treatment. However, in France, where statistics have been carefully kept and where acupuncture is an acceptable form of therapy, the recoveries reported have been excellent.

In the Chinese culture, a doctor who waited for a patient to become ill before giving treatment was a poor doctor indeed. The Chinese pay their doctors to keep them well, not merely to treat them when they are sick:

> ...to administer medicines to diseases which have already developed...is comparable to the behavior of those persons who begin to dig a well after they have become thirsty...[2]

The use of pulse diagnosis is founded on the belief that many days, months, even years pass before a disease shows itself. Some symptoms are discernable and will register in an abnormality of the pulse. By palpation of these pulses, the traditional practitioner reportedly is able to discern which part of the body is malfunctioning. A patient who sees the acupuncturist every six months, or once every year for the exceptionally healthy, will find that overall well-being can be maintained at a high level.

Chinese therapists admit that in our modern civilization it is difficult to completely avoid threats to our health and well-being. However, people born healthy, of healthy parents, infrequently become sick and are cured more quickly if they care for themselves.

Cooperating with your acupuncturist and getting the proper amount of exercise, healthful food and relaxation will help you live a pain-free and long life.

Shiatsu[3]

If you are dead set against trying acupuncture, another option is Shiatsu (pronounced shee-AT-soo). Shiatsu is the manipulative (hand pressure) method of dealing with some of the same problems addressed by acupuncture. Diseases treated by Shiatsu should be in elementary stages. The treatment is slower, but if you stay with it, you will find relief if acupuncture could have helped you.

The many books on the subject give explanations as well as drawings of where to exert pressure. They also explain the circular method of pressing the fingers.

The practitioner uses the balls of the thumbs and palms of the hands to exert pressure at points on the body to contribute to the healing process. Using the innate powers of self-healing, the body is encouraged to repair its own problem areas with the help of digital pressure.

Serious illnesses require the care of a professional Shiatsu practitioner who has studied human anatomy, massage and Shiatsu techniques. You can take care of fatigue, aching shoulders, backache and toothache yourself by following the charts offered. The circular motions of the thumb and palm stimulate the body and create additional circulation at the point of pressure and prevent congestion in other parts of the body. The pressure must *never* exceed more than three seconds in one spot around the neck because injury or death may result, but pressure may be applied as long as five to seven seconds elsewhere. Using a chart to guide you, press each of the indicated points firmly but not hurtfully. This may be done even when you are taking a bath.

Fatigue, which can accumulate without your realizing it until you are near exhaustion, may be dispelled with Shiatsu pressure treatment.

The main advantages of the Shiatsu method are that you can put it to immediate use and apply the treatment yourself. The treatment takes only minutes and you can maintain it easily by yourself as a supplement to the everyday general care of your body.

Professional Shiatsu experts should be consulted before long-term therapy for chronic conditions is considered. Some professional Shiatsu experts work with the medical profession.

There are no harmful or unpleasant side effects with this treatment, and the body is encouraged to help itself in harmony with nature. The fact that it requires no tools and can be done alone makes it an ideal treatment for the elderly. Once the present malfunction is under control, a few minutes of Shiatsu treatment morning and night can keep one in good health.[4] Try it!

Nutrition Therapy

Although over-worked, depleted soil can not produce good cotton or wheat, doctors rarely consider the quality of the farming soil when they insist that foods will provide all the vitamins and minerals needed. Earth starved for fertilizers, minerals, or water is bound to produce food low in essential qualities. A doctor who says you do not need vitamins because you can get the required food values from the food you eat every day, does not know the quality of the foods you are buying in the supermarket or how they are prepared. The doctor may not know a great deal about nutrition and may assume that if s/he does not know it, it is not important.

Another problem is the individual diet. People on-the-run who settle for a hamburger, a batch of french fries, and a soft drink are getting calories, some vitamins and some minerals, but are they getting sufficient nutrients for their needs? The person who lifts cement blocks for a living certainly needs a different diet from the desk-bound accountant, although they might know each other and meet over a hamburger and beer.

Food additives have been supplementing our food for years to discourage vermin from eating the products in storage. These additives may not be healthful and often provide the counter-balance for necessary nutrients.

A food additive is a chemical that is added by the manufacturer to make the food more attractive to the buyer, to change the color to a more acceptable one, or to preserve the product on the shelf for long periods of time. Estimates are that hundreds of chemicals are added to our foods. Some even attempt to replace the vitamins and minerals bleached, washed, and cooked out of them. Synthetic foods are made to look and taste like real foods, and thickeners help keep foods together so that they are easily handled or used.

Although the Food and Drug Administration supervises the use of chemicals added to our foods and is required to ban any additive that has proved damaging to laboratory animals, officials make no attempt to evaluate the cumulative effect of any drug or chemical used. Some drugs pass out of the system with the other waste products of the body, but many others do not. They have a tendency to collect in various parts of the body, so that over a period of time they may cause serious damage.

For instance, older people are particularly vulnerable to the dangers inherent in aluminum poisoning, but their symptoms of confusion and mental deterioration are passed off as part of the aging process. It might be revealing to test for the symptoms of aluminum poisoning, according to Dr. Armand Lione, writing in *Perspectives on Aging*.[5]

No evaluations of how much aluminum is acceptable in the diet exist, but the list of products we eat that contain aluminum in some form is frighteningly long: cake mixes, frozen doughs, pancake mixes, some self-rising flours, processed cheese and "cheese foods"—especially those sold individually sliced and wrapped. Sodium aluminum phosphate, also referred to as "alum," is contained in many household baking powders. In fact, it may comprise as much as 21 to 26 percent of the content of the baking powder.

Some brands of commercially prepared pickles are made with ammonium or potassium aluminum sulphates. Aluminum silicates are commonly used and may consist of up to 2.0 percent of the dry powdered non-dairy creamers. Incidentally, some chewing gums contain substantial amounts of aluminum. Non-prescription drugs such as antacids, buffered aspirin, anti-diarrheal products, douches, and hemorrhoidal medications may have considerable amounts of aluminum in them, as do many anti-perspirants and lipsticks.

Acid-type foods cooked in aluminum could release as much as four milligrams of aluminum to *each serving*. Acidic beverages such as coffee brewed in aluminum cookware may be a great source of aluminum intake. Some elderly people who have died after long hospitalizations from Alzheimer's disease have shown huge accumulations of aluminum in the brain tissues.

Nutritious diets consisting of plenty of fresh fruits and vegetables, a good amount of pure water, a lifestyle free of the influences of tobacco, food additives, coloring matter, chemicals, and other pollutants, give the immune system of the body the stimulation it needs to fight disease. In the case of cancer, for instance, immunotherapy in the form of BCG (Bacillus Calmette-Guerin) vaccine along with gamma globulin and proper nutrition and diet sometimes arrest the disease. If it cannot, it will strengthen patients receiving traditional therapy so that the noxious side-effects will be less of a problem.

In a 1984 conference, the Livingston-Wheeler Foundation of San Diego presented the theory that cancer is caused by a microbe, is infectious but pleomorphic—has many shapes or crystallizes into many forms. Is cleaning up our food supply and immunotherapy the answer to cancer?

Cancer research is one of the largest industries in the United States today. At least twelve billion dollars of tax money and contributions have gone into the accumulation of information about chemotherapy and radiation as treatment for cancer, but Dr. Owen Webster feels these may do more harm than good.[6] Immunotherapy, if properly used to arrest the disease, could save many lives, he advises. Dr. Lewis Thomas, author, physician, and president of Sloane-Kettering says:

> . . . . much of what is done in the treatment of cancer by surgery, radi-
> ation, chemotherapy, represents "half-way technology". . . directed at
> the existence of already-established cancer. . . but not at the mech-
> anisms by which cells become neoplastic (neo-meaning new; plastic-
> meaning contributing to building tissues) . . . (and) if nothing is done
> to build up an immunity, there will be a recurrence of cancer. . .[7]

Dr. Livingston-Wheeler believes cancer is preventable and probably curable right now. Over two hundred million children in China have been vaccinated with BCG vaccine and work will soon be done to evaluate their resistance to cancer, leukemia, and tuberculosis. In Chicago, approximately 20,000 babies were vaccinated with BCG vaccine and gamma globulin and twenty years later were compared to an even larger number of unvaccinated children. An 85 percent drop in the mortality rate from leukemia and a 74 percent drop in all forms of cancer were discovered.[8]

To learn more about this immunotherapy program, you may contact The Livingston-Wheeler Medical Clinic, 3233 Duke Street, San Diego, CA 92110.

Nutritionists can help to plan a diet designed especially for you, taking into account your body-style and structure, your needs in relation to how you exert yourself during the day, and what you do for recreation.

Each person is born with a constitution different from anyone else's. Because one person does very well on a vegetarian diet does not mean this diet will suit someone else. Another person might be the kind who digests vegetables at top speed and becomes hungry an hour after eating a vegetarian meal.[9] For this kind of person, food must contain hard-to-digest materials such as animal meat and/or fats to last until the next meal. Most of us require both vegetables and meat to feel full and able to wait for the next meal.

"Minimum daily requirements" has no meaning in this context. What is your "minimum" might be a "maximum" to the person working right beside you. When supplementing any nutritional regimen you should consider the kind of food that will assist in retaining your own good health.

Your weight reflects the balance between calories ingested and calories consumed by the body. This balance depends on age, hormones, genetic background, and exercise. If you go right from a big meal and sit down for several hours, the unneeded calories will pile up and you will deposit fat cells in places where they will be hard to work off. The same meal will be worked off by heavy physical labor, however, such as lifting cement blocks or house-building. Your body should be properly tuned for the work and play it does, and you—not anyone else—must see that it is.

There have been stunning discoveries of the importance of a proper diet. In a fairly recent edition of *Medical News*, a front-page story headlined "Supplement Boosts I.Q. in Retarded" detailed the fact that ". . . mentally retarded children showed surprising and dramatic improvement in I.Q., growth and visual acuity after receiving a special nutritional supplement of minerals and vitamins in an eight-months' trial . . . ."[10]

Children identified as having behavior problems are often displaying a sensitivity to food additives. Studies show that when their diets are altered so that they are not exposed to food additives, they behave as normal children.

Once in a while in a letter-to-the-editor column of the newspaper, you get a heart-warming reassurance that people are learning the importance of nutrition. One woman wrote that she "stumbled across a doctor who is also a nutritionist," and ended seven years of torment for herself, her husband, and her thirteen-year-old son. For seven years her son had been prescribed drugs to alter his behavior, without doctors making an attempt to find the cause. The nutritionist-doctor, using cytotoxic blood tests, revealed sensitivity to the foods that were making her son unbalanced, depending upon whether he had had his medication that day. Now he is a normal boy—on a restricted diet.[11]

For twenty-five years or more, cattle have been fed female sex hormones to encourage them to grow larger, fatter, more meaty. Although it has not been determined whether the presence of these additional female sex hormones has had an influence on our children and their health, the FDA has tried to ban this practice from time to time.

Whose responsibility is it to do the research on the hundreds of food additives in our diet? What about the cooking utensils made of aluminum and the effects of refined carbohydrates? Data that reveal test results often are not available to the general public.

The news media is controlled by the corporations that advertise in their pages, buy air time on television and radio and pay heavily for the space in the magazines we read. These are the same corporations responsible for our foods and the food additives that go into them, the contamination of our air and the illnesses that this brings, and the production of medications that are becoming more suspect all the time. Sadly enough, these companies and institutions do not act on knowledge and research findings independently. They wait until the pressure of public opinion forces them to do so.[12]

A nutritionist, homeopathic physician, chiropractor, or osteopath who also practices in the field of "wholistic" (or holistic) medicine, including nutrition, can help you design the diet applicable to your own health and happiness. This person will outline the methods of cooking, the amounts to eat, and the fresh fruits, vegetables, and pure water that will keep your body in good repair. Let one of these people help you get the best combination of foods into your diet so that your body may heal itself.

Osteopathy[13]

Founded by Dr. Andrew Taylor Still in the late 1800s, osteopathy is based upon the interdependence of all the parts of the body and the need to treat all parts of the body without regard for the specific location of the symptoms. Using the built-in repair processes of the body, the circulatory system is encouraged to provide integrating functions for self-regulation and self-healing through manipulative (hand) therapy with a resort to surgical intervention only if considered more suitable.

Because of the definition of "disease" as seen in the discipline of osteopathy, Dr. Still taught that alteration of any structure of the body causes abnormalities. When that happens, the blood supply changes, and the entire body finds itself in a state of "dis-ease" or illness.

Osteopathy is principally concerned with the spine as the basis of correct treatment and alignment. Osteopaths feel that spinal arthritis (spondyolitis), for instance, is not inevitable in elderly patients, but can be treated and the painful effects reversed by correct adjustment of the inflamed joint or joints which releases the pressure on the nervous system. Then the organs of the body can be influenced toward good health.

The courses of preparation to become an osteopath include the same four years of medical training and the same licensing examinations required for other physicians. As a matter of fact, the American Medical Association would prefer combining the two schools of practice, although the American Osteopathic Association continues to reaffirm its interest in staying independent.

While the total number of doctors in the United States has increased by 95 percent in the last four decades, the proportion of general practitioners has gone down from 74 percent to 21 percent. Osteopathy has been filling the need for old-fashioned family physicians. Osteopaths have consented to settle in non-urban areas where few doctors have agreed to locate. An earlier dispute over the medical credentials of osteopaths was resolved by an American Medical Association investigation into their educational preparation. The AMA discovered that the training given at osteopathic colleges and medical schools was not significantly different from the training given at standard medical colleges.

There are well-documented cases of conditions considered mental or emotional in origin being cured by osteopathic manipulation. While Dr. Still worked with patients to increase intake of oxygen and to correct the alignment of vertebrae and organs, he required that people also correct their dietary deficiencies as well.

Although the majority of patients arrive at the office of the osteopath with spinal problems, the doctor of osteopathy can deal with problems of a much wider nature without the use of drugs. Often the patient has turned to osteopathy as a last resort, after having made the rounds of medical practitioners who have failed to arrest, no less cure, the condition. The patient and the doctor together must face the possibility that even osteopathy cannot help the condition if it has gone on too long, and the deterioration has been too severe.

In many parts of the country, osteopaths have assisted with births, either in hospitals or in patients' homes. Osteopathy has produced many successful deliveries and, in more than one instance, pre-birth treatment helped to make the delivery easy and almost pain-free.

This is one of the largest of the healing sciences outside the area of the orthodoxy of allopathic medicine. Osteopathy has a good track record in helping the sick body to restore good health and smooth functioning without drugs.

Chiropractic[14]

In southwestern France cave paintings have been found depicting spinal adjustments such as those being used in chiropractic today. It is estimated that these paintings were done at least 17,500 years before Christ. In the fourth and fifth centuries Hippocrates wrote several treatises on spinal articulation, and spinal manipulation was practiced by Chinese, Japanese, and Tibetans in Asia. The Native Americans of Mexico, Central and North America have practiced forms of spinal manipulation, as their paintings and artifacts reveal.

The practitioners of chiropractic medicine attempt to restore the integrity of the nervous system and organize the body to enable it to return to normal functioning through the "effective use of hands." Their belief in holistic medicine, the treatment of the entire patient instead of the symptoms in a particular part of the body, makes chiropractic an acceptable form of therapy in the suburban and rural areas in which many have chosen to practice. The chiropractor often takes the place of the family doctor, and the relationship with the patient and the family are quite personal.

Chiropractic's founder in the United States, Daniel David Palmer, based his belief on manipulation of the body through the spinal cord's nerves and nerve impulses that send messages to the rest of the body. Most of the patients who seek chiropractic help, however, complain of back, arm, or leg pain. While patients with internal problems usually see a general practitioner or specialist, others have found that the record of assistance with nerve or spine problems in standard Western medicine has left much to be desired. Back and limb injuries and problems have had a tendency to rise in the last couple of decades as more leisure leads to greater participation in sports. This has given chiropractic an opportunity to prove its value.

In some instances chiropractors have supplemented their manipulative treatments with mechanical aids developed recently, although the basic treatment itself is contained in the "laying on of hands." The training and education of chiropractors—while different from that of osteopaths and physicians—takes six years of college study and internship, and the areas studied are pertinent to primary health care. Although the greatest number of practitioners go into general practice, some individuals specialize in such fields as athletic injuries and industrial or insurance problems. Certification has already been established in roentgenology (the branch of radiology which deals with the use of x-rays) and orthopedics.

The chiropractic philosophy is that the secret of health is lost when we try to effect a cure without discovering the cause of the illness. Practitioners feel that drugs prevent the flow of health and that people should not take them. Practitioners find that patients generally have explored and employed traditional methods and found them unable to help before they come to a chiropractor.

> . . .We throw off our belief in saints; a trust in St. Erasmus for stomach ailments; St. Anastosias for diseases of the throat . . . but we have other "shrines"—pharmaceutical cartels with experimental remedies more hazardous to those with psychogenic ills than hopeful prayers and the laying on of hands could ever be. . .[15]

Adjustment of the disorders of the locomotion system such as joints are supplemented by adjustments, exercise, and nutritional guidance. Shoes are examined; sitting, standing, bed and work postures are carefully evaluated and changes are recommended so that treatments will help the patients as soon as possible. This will help to sustain progress toward better health and prevent the recurrence of the problem.

The differences between chiropractic and osteopathy may not seem very clear. Both seem to treat the same types of complaints, and both treat patients with a "hands-on" form of therapy. The origins of both methods are the chief sources of alienation. Dr. Still, the founder of osteopathy, believed that the blood supply (unimpeded circulation) was the basic component for health. Dr. Palmer's emphasis was on the nervous system. However, both branches of manipulative healing have their own established organizations and will probably continue to be independent of each other. If they should ever unite, they would surely create a formidable front for the release of healing therapies from the tight control of the medical professionals.

Herbal Medicine

The use of herbs in healing has a venerable history. Written records marked on papyrus go back at least to 2,000 B.C. In primitive cultures, medicine men or women concocted remedies from the wild plants in their environment, and the efficacy of these treatments was always emphatically proclaimed. We know today that faith in the eventual recovery is more than half the battle when you are ailing.

Recipes and directions for the use of these herbal remedies come from ancient, hand-copied manuscripts and may be viewed in museums in Greece where monks are said to use them still in preparing medicines today. Many superstitions surround the use of herbs in food as well as medicine. The most prominent of them has been the "Doctrine of Signatures," which indicated that the value of an herb was directly related to the organ of the body that the shape or color of the herb resembled. If the plant was shaped like a lung, the herb was able to cure problems related to the lungs; if the stems or leaves were red, it was claimed that the blood would benefit from the herb.

The herbal offerings of the Native Americans, however, were superior to those offered by European-trained doctors early in our history, although the American colonists did bring herbs with them when they came to the New World.

In the Orient, the use of herbs for healing continues today. In Sri Lanka this practice is called Ayurvedic Medicine, and in India and China it is called Oriental Medicine. The origin of the formulas is buried in the distant past, but is claimed to be at least three thousand years old. Vaccination, anesthesia by inhalation, and diet as a cure for illness are traced back this far, but only a few of these techniques have been adopted by Western medicine in the last hundred years or so. Surgery, too, was a developed science in those early days. Records show that cataracts were removed and cosmetic surgery (mainly on the nose) was performed in addition to the dietary and herbal remedies for sickness.

Training in herbal or Ayurvedic Medicine is through recitation and repetition with a considerable amount of practice through an apprenticeship with an older established practitioner.

Through the years what has remained the same in the treatment called Ayurveda has been the importance of the Tridosha, or three elements: air, water, and fire. It is the Ayurvedic belief that all the areas of human function can fit into one of these "doshas." The physician's primary task is to observe the patient's behavior and attitude and then make an analysis by dividing observations into one of the two groups: the group that controls the internal senses or the group that controls the external senses. Knowing the patient's age, nationality, family life and circumstances, the physician can proceed to formulate a therapy.

Treatment for illness analyzes which of the three elements of the person needs treatment. When that is determined, the other two elements of the body are encouraged to stimulation and good health. Foods that arouse the third or sickly portion of the body are curtailed, and the diet then is tried for a while before any medicine is prescribed. In this way the patient does not have to suffer from being ill as well as from a wrong choice of medication. Practitioners know that some herbs would not work with some people, and different people would require different herbs.

The physician practicing Ayurveda not only advises the patient during times of illness, but also guides the person during times of good health. The physician is responsible for creating a diet especially for the patient, assisting in the regulation of personal habits, even assisting in the choice of a marital partner and advising on sexual behavior. Since the patient's religious faith is likely to be the same or have the same roots as the doctor's, the doctor is also the counselor in the spiritual sphere.

The herbs dispensed are divided into several categories; some are considered hot and some cold by their very nature, and to this day they are chosen with a particular patient in mind.

In our culture, fewer and fewer people grew the herbs that kept the old-fashioned folk medicines alive, and soon the pharmaceutical companies began to produce synthetics as substitutes for the old herbal remedies. People stopped growing simple herbs for their food, even though they were easy to grow and could be used with little, if any, processing. Herbs are plants that are not woody, but die back to a rootstock in the winter. Nothing in the modern pharmacopoeia can produce some of the wonderful aromas, seasonings, or time-tested treatments of long ago. Many natural food stores have the herbs necessary for healthful teas, poultices, or ointments for curative concoctions, but some you will have to grow for yourself. Such is the case with aloe vera, for instance, a treatment for burns which is superior to the medications offered on the market through prescriptions or over-the-counter. Aloe vera is also less expensive.

Preparing herbs for medicinal purposes is rarely a complicated process. Most often the herb is not boiled but just added to already boiled water. The container is then carefully covered, and the preparation left to steep three, ten, or twenty minutes. Sometimes it is necessary to leave the concoction overnight.

The discovery of penicillin highlighted the fact that herbal medicine needed to be reexamined and rediscovered. Healers of many cultures used bread or bread-making doughs, wrapped them around a piece of copper, producing the mold that gave us penicillin. Then the development of antibiotics took off, following the path that penicillin had shown.

Herbs brought from all over the world are being examined for their healing potential. India produces the basic plant from which tranquilizers are being made today—rawolfia or reserpine is being used in the treatment of mental distress. A huge amount of work remains to be done in assessing the value of the quarter- to half-million herbs still untested from all over the globe. The contributions these herbs may make might astound us.

Yes, the importance of herbs is again being recognized. People are starting to use simpler foods, adding herbs and spices to dress them up in place of additives available on the food store shelves. People are discovering that there are herbs to enliven you, herbs to depress the appetite, herbs to sooth and relax you, and herbs to recall the delicious European or Asiatic foods tasted overseas.

Not all herbs are useable in all forms, however. Some herbs are dangerous if served in large quantities or if cooked. Others are safe enough to eat cooked, but the juices left after they are cooked are poisonous. Read carefully and learn about any herb you decide to use. The ones you grow from seed available in the United States can be researched in almost any public library.

Care must be taken before self-medication with herbs is attempted. You might use a preparation that will be harmful instead of useful, if not used in the right quantities, or not carefully applied. You should consult an authority on herbal medicine, but if you cannot locate one nearby, consult several books on the subject from the nearest public library.

Using herbs, fresh or dried, on your food on a regular basis is a healthful and flavorful practice. It also adds to the nutriments we take in every day and may help to make drugs unnecessary.

Exercises

If chiropractic and/or osteopathy has been helpful to you, you may benefit from properly chosen consistent exercises which will help you to stay in good physical condition. Exercise will keep in place the adjustments made by the manipulations of the chiropractor or osteopath.

Properly-trained gymnastic supervisors can help you select exercises that will, almost from the beginning, give you a feeling of well-being. In addition you should concentrate on building up the muscles in the areas of stress. Easy, warm-up exercises should be used to start a program each time you go to the gym. They can also be done at home, but often people find it difficult to follow a regular regimen on their own. It is important to find the time every day for keeping muscles in good tone and for strengthening the body structure.

Each period of assessment will give the gym supervisor and you an opportunity to evaluate the progress you have made. You will have a chance to cancel some of the program or change the emphasis if needed. You will be amazed at the difference in your pep and vigor, your arising in the morning, and your ability to sleep through the night.

Find the kind and amount of exercise that is right for you and then go to it, but bear in mind the following:

—Choose all-round exercises for at least some portion of the regimen, something that will stretch the arms, the body and the legs.

—Choose to do the kind of exercise you like the most: a game of tennis or croquet on the lawn. Everyone should play a little.

—Choose one or two exercises that you can use to check your progress: can you do more sit-ups, can you touch your toes one more time?

—Some of the exercises should be ones that you can do alone and at home. Even on days that you can't get to the gym, you will have a group of exercises planned that will give you an extra little boost toward getting to the work of the day. There is a group of people who are trying, particularly in California, to establish a connection between the "inner self" and sports, with the hope that there will be a useful therapy developed for psychological as well as physical well-being.

A word of caution! You can't undo years of neglect in a week, ten days, or even a month. Building up to a fairly comprehensive exercise program should be done slowly and under the jurisdiction of a caring and knowledgeable individual trained for the job.

Reflexology

Little is certain about the origins of reflexology, but it is known to have been used by natives of Kenya and by some Native American tribes. Early in this century, a Dr. Fitzgerald used the method in the United States as a form of anesthesia for small operations or for the pain during childbirth. At that time it was called "zone therapy."

Eunice Ingham and her nephew, Dwight C. Byers, currently director of the International Institute of Reflexology, brought this therapy to the attention of the public. The philosophy of reflexology is fairly similar to that of medicine in general and alternative therapies in particular: the body must be brought back to a state of homeostasis (home-ee-oh-STAY-sis, equilibrium) if the patient is ill or just not feeling well. Every part of the body must be in harmony and the intricate workings of the whole being must be adjusted and soothed.

The methods seem simple and, with a little effort, could probably be learned by the patient or a member of the family who would like to help. Hands and thumbs are used to massage the reflexes that are present in the feet, which link up with all parts of the body. A tender place in some area of either foot indicates a problem with the particular part of the body related to that reflex. The more tender the spot, the more serious is the condition.

Releasing tensions is the basic reason for the need of therapy. Massaging the feet encourages a full supply of blood to ailing areas in distress. The energy that is sent to the spot revitalizes the entire body and solves over three-quarters of the problems brought to the therapist. These problems revolve around nervous tension.

If the feet cannot be worked on, the hands have the same reflexes and may be used for treatment. The cross-reflexes in the shoulder, hip, elbow and knee that work with the feet and hands are particularly valuable in difficult cases. If the illness has been developing over a period of time, the recovery will be a gradual process. However, the outlook and appearance of many patients have changed and improved after just a few treatments, regardless of their ages.

Although there is an effort to discover where the body needs attention by finding tenderness in the foot, the patient experiences little, if any, pain connected with the treatments. No gadgets or equipment are involved. Only hands are used for the treatment.

Reflexology is useful for the type of circulation troubles encountered by older people. Where patients have been doing poorly under other forms of treatment, it is possible to make another start with reflexology.

If you want to find a reflexologist in your area, the International Institute of Reflexology, P.O. Box 12642, St. Petersburg, FL 33733 will be glad to help.

Homeopathy[16]

This form of therapy was discovered by Dr. Samuel C. Hahnemann in the early 1800s. After finishing his medical training, he practiced medicine for a while. The methods he saw for treating illnesses seemed brutal and senseless; the bleeding, the purging and cauterizing were, he felt, interfering with the body's own ability to heal itself. Dr. Hahnemann was denounced as a heretic by the rest of the medical establishment and found it necessary to do medical translation to make a living. Through this translation work he came across the data that led him to adopt the form of therapy known as homeopathy.

As a healthy individual, Dr. Hahnemann took some quinine and produced symptoms that looked, felt and acted like malaria. He concluded that small quantities of quinine would relieve malarial symptoms and proceeded to prove that it did.

With the help of friends and well-wishers, he proved, or supervised the proving of, ninety-nine substances that alleviated illnesses by the time he died at the age of eighty-eight. Hahnemann's followers added six hundred other medicines to the homeopathic pharmacopoeia by the early 1900s. Dr. Hahnemann wrote four major works in the field of medicine and laid down specific rules regarding the preparation and prescription of the remedies he had developed. These rules are still used today.

Basically, the theory of homeopathy is that disease is an aberration from the state of health and "like heals like." Dr. Hahnemann taught that an herb, medicine or remedy can cure an illness if, when that substance is given to a well individual, it produces the same symptoms displayed by the sick person. In other words, if you should develop a fever with the usual symptoms of flushed face, rapid heart beat, dilated pupils, and a general feeling of unwellness, the homeopathic physician will search through the pharmacopoeia for a remedy that, under the condition it is given to a well individual, produces the same sort of symptoms. That medicine will cure the fever if given in very small doses to the sick person. The minimum doses given to the patient do not contain enough matter to act directly on the tissues. The medication is non-toxic and has no side effects. Only one medication is given at a time so that one drug will not work against another or make another drug more virulent. Practitioners of homeopathy are proud that in 150 years of this type of treatment, not a single medication they use has ever had to be recalled.

Doctors who practiced homeopathy were licensed medical practitioners, educated in the orthodox methods of the day, who had "defected" to this more humane method.

All homeopathic medicines are prepared almost entirely from fresh materials, made into a "mother tincture" and stored for use. When needed, the correct and smallest possible dosage is prescribed and mixed with a neutral material such as pure alcohol, water, or sugar. The mixture is shaken rapidly in a special manner and it is sometimes made into small tablets. The small size of the dose will not aggravate the illness.

Resurgence of interest in natural healing methods may signify a revolt against the widespread use of dangerous drugs prescribed in allopathic (orthodox) medicine. Homeopathy is more acceptable elsewhere in the world. The royal family of England has been treated with homeopathic medicine since the time of Queen Victoria, and homeopathic medical colleges may be found in London, Glasgow, India, Mexico and South America.

The principles of homeopathy are simple but effective:

1. The doctor will spend enough time with each patient to listen carefully to the list of symptoms, and determine the nature of the patient's emotional and mental state.

2. Treatments cost less and require fewer visits because the patients' abilities to heal themselves are encouraged and enhanced. Patients become ill less often as a result of the treatments.

3. Little need exists for laboratory tests and x-rays since the homeopathic physician believes the "life force" changes can be noted long before measurable changes occur in blood or tissues. The time the therapist takes discussing symptoms with you will reveal the changes in the "life forces." This will consequently result in earlier turn-around.

4. The patient may purchase a kit to treat a number of illnesses. The twenty-eight remedies the kit contains are carefully designated and explained. In this way, patients are encouraged to be responsible for their own health problems.

5. Homeopathic remedies do not have side-effects. About five hundred remedies are in common use in homeopathy, and the firms that supply the materials for the concoctions have been doing so since the mid-1900s. The materials are clean, pure, and reliable each time you use them.

In the event you want to find a homeopathic physician in your area, communicate with the National Center for Homeopathy, 1500 Massachusetts Ave. N.W., Suite 41, Washington, DC 20005 or the American Center for Homeopathy, 6560 Backlick Road, Suite 211, Springfield VA 22150. They will also be glad to help you find a center close by that will supply you with a kit of homeopathic remedies.

Yoga

Yoga has been practiced since 3,000 B.C. The various systems that make up Yoga have been designed and practiced throughout the years for the development of human potential. Yoga has nothing to do with caste, religion, or any particular nation. It does not espouse a particular God, nor does it deny the existence of God.

Hatha Yoga is concerned primarily with the physical aspect of our being, and requires the use of many postures and body attitudes which must be taught to the aspiring practitioner in slow stages. This form of Yoga has attracted the interest of the Western world.

Yoga disciplines the mind and the body through self-study and self-knowledge to maintain perfect health through mental, moral, physical, and spiritual training. It offers people resistance to disease, a beautiful body, longevity, and mental and spiritual sublimation. The concentration is on the body and its health. You are encouraged to meditate on one portion of the body—the tip of the nose or the middle of the forehead—to become more intensely aware of the workings of your body and achieve extraordinary power over yourself.

Instruction in Hatha Yoga is available in the United States not only in specialized environments, but exercise classes and YM- or YWCAs often have sessions for teaching the breathing and posture program.

Yoga does not require violent or exhausting exercises. In fact, to begin you should get into an easy, relaxed position. The postures themselves are geometric shapes and represent vital centers characteristic of living and inanimate objects. Practicing these postures even ten minutes a day will be beneficial, but it takes perhaps two or three weeks to learn the basic exercises that should be practiced throughout your life. The exercises—for both men and women—make the body flexible and improve the coordination between mind and body. With practice you should be able to increase the amount of time you can remain in the posture. The exercises should be done in a well-ventilated room and on a rug, mattress, or blanket stretched on the floor.

Many books are available in paperback and hard-cover, outlining the exercises and the philosophy of Yoga. Yoga will teach the student how to keep the glands of the body in excellent condition and tune up the nerve-force that helps the spine preserve its flexibility. Advocates of Yoga feel that cancer, heart disease, and mental disorders may be brought under control or prevented through elimination of impurities, by resting different parts of the body consciously as well as unconsciously. You can rejuvenate organs that have deteriorated by sending cosmic energy to them through meditation, and by decreasing the amount of energy used by the body through learning how to relax the mind and the body. A good book for the beginner is *Integral Yoga Hatha* by Yogiraj Sri Swami Satchadananda, published by Holt, Rinehart and Winston in 1970.

Laying On of Hands (Therapeutic Touch)

Throughout history, writings, songs and stories have told of men or women who could heal by the process of laying on of hands. As being taught today, the laying on of hands has not really changed in concept from the depiction of it on the walls of caves estimated to be up to 15,000 years old. The practice was used in India, China, Egypt and then moved into Western Europe during the Middle Ages. Church histories of that period document episodes of the laying on of hands.

The Sanskrit term for this healing is "prana," or—as closely as we can translate the term—"human energy transfer." Believed to be the force behind the life process itself, prana could be described as the unique power responsible for healing and regeneration.

In our scientific age when all processes are open to doubt, this form of healing has met with exclamations of "quackery!" But there is little doubt that some people do have the ability to alter ailing conditions of people by approaching and lifting the hands toward the sick individual and by concentrating on the person as long as fifteen minutes.

The laying on of hands, as taught and used in this country today, is referred to as "Therapeutic Touch." Teachers and practitioners claim that almost everyone has the potential for developing this ability. It is merely necessary to learn to concentrate carefully and intensely in order to learn to play the role of healer, so that the flow of energy in plentiful supply in you may be made available to the person in need of such help.

For those ailing and in need of healing, the freedom from intrusion into the body and the fact that little inconvenience is connected with having someone work on you make it well worth a try. Therapeutic touch relaxes you subtly and reduces the pain, providing your ailing body with the spur needed to continue the healing processes. The hands of the healer are cupped and gently extended, resting about half an inch from the part of the body to be treated. Afterward, patients report a feeling of release and well-being and a surge of energy that gives a feeling that relief of the illness is imminent.

Therapeutic touch has been used for abdominal cramps, headaches, and even to soothe a crying baby. A good book on the subject is *The Therapeutic Touch: How to Use Your Hands to Help or to Heal* by Dolores Krieger, published in 1979 by Prentice-Hall.

This ancient but simple method of healing may be the answer to your own or someone else's healing process and is worth exploring.

Massage[17]

Massage is a method of treating the body for remedial or hygienic purposes, consisting of rubbing, stroking, kneading, or tapping with the hand or an instrument. The medical dictionary adds the caution that the massage must always be applied upon the bare skin.

The purpose of massage is to make you feel better, more relaxed, and to relieve pressure when physical activity has been prolonged. Stress can develop in many ways such as having to stand in one place to work or having to sit in a wheelchair. This type of treatment may range from massage of the eardrum membrane to the emergency use of massage to restore the heartbeat when it has stopped. This technique is done by putting pressure on the heart for short periods of time to force the blood out of the heart so that the release of pressure will allow the blood to return, as if the heart were beating.

Electrovibrators are often used for massage purposes when large portions of the body are in need of stimulation. The type of treatment known as "general massage" involves a head-to-toe kneading program, starting with the toes and feet and extending toward the head. This therapy takes about thirty or forty minutes and consists of short upward rotary movements. The patient is covered at all times, except for the portion of the body being massaged. This is the most common and most appealing form of massage and is often an accompaniment to a Turkish bath. Massage is not considered therapy, except in the sense that it provides a form of relaxation.

For the specialized kind of massage of hydrotherapy or hydropneumatic massage, specific equipment is required. Air is forced through a tube, at the end of which is a chamber containing water. The water chamber is applied to the part of the body being massaged.

When the ailing part of the body is internal, massage by kneading, stroking or rubbing as close to the painful or afflicted area is often helpful. A type of massage called tremolo massage is applied in an off-and-then-on manner that gives a feeling of interrupted pressures. This is excellent for stimulating circulation.

In India and Sri Lanka, mothers establish a special bond with their babies through the art of exquisitely gentle massage. They describe it as using their hands softly and smoothly to replace the feeling of protection the baby lost when it was born, the reinforcement for the back, the warm fluidity of its surroundings. This is practiced by sitting on the floor so that the legs, either with or without a soft warm towel over them, can touch the back and upper legs of the child. The mother will apply oil to her hands and to the chest of the baby, then stroke down the legs of the baby, maintaining a slow and rhythmic tempo. The rest of the body is massaged gently, one arm at a time, then the wrists and fingers are gently kneaded. Then the baby is turned over and gently stroked. Then comes the bath, warm and reassuring, as the mother allows the delicate body to float. This removes whatever is left of tension and hunger for protection. In the Far East, this is considered a dialogue of love upon which to base the tender relationship for the rest of life.

Birthing

Alternatives to hospital deliveries are becoming more appealing and available. Homelike birthing rooms are becoming more common in hospitals across the country, and the formidable, brightly-lit, cold, and austere hospital labor rooms are going out of fashion. Many women are abandoning the stark severity of hospital labor rooms for home deliveries, making it necessary for hospitals to create a more welcoming atmosphere.

Childbirth programs are being developed all over the country that involve the father and, if the couple desires it, other members of the family. Midwife-assisted births were common for centuries before doctors established the concept that birthing was a pathological experience. Women today are attempting to return this experience to the joyful, family-oriented occasion it used to be.

Recent trends in childbirth include underwater delivery. In this, the baby remains connected to the umbilical cord, safe from having to breathe the atmosphere until it is brought out into the warmed air and wrapped in a blanket.

Alternatives to hospital care are developing in many other directions as well, all with the intent to dispense with elements that interfere with the fullest appreciation of the event. All methods give great consideration to the safety and comfort of both the baby and the mother.

Followers of alternative birthing methods feel that the absence of harsh lights, monitoring gadgets and forceps leads to emotionally healthier children and closer bonds between the parents and the baby.

This new listing on the subject might be of interest: *Directory of Alternate Birth Services,* National Association of Parents and Professionals for Safe Alternatives in Childbirth, 2nd edition, available from the International Association of Parents and Professionals for Safe Alternatives in Childbirth, P.O. Box 428, Marble Hill, MO 63764.

If you still feel your problems have not been addressed, you have one more resource available. A non-profit, tax-exempt clearing house for health information called the Association for Medical and Health Alternatives (AMHA) is available to do research for individuals at a nominal sum. They will clarify diagnoses, suggest alternative forms of therapy, and tell you where to go for further information. They plan to publish books on specific health problems in the near future. For more information, write to the Association for Medical and Health Alternatives, P.O. Box 112, Clearwater, FL 33517.

The *Holistic Health Handbook,* published by the Berkeley Holistic Center in California, is another excellent source book that describes many alternative modalities of healing.

NOTES

1. Felix Mann, *Acupuncture, The Chinese Art of Healing and How It Works Scientifically* and Toguchi Masaru, *The Complete Guide to Acupuncture.*
2. Toguchi Masaru, *The Complete Guide to Acupuncture,* p. 14.
3. Toru Namikoshi, *Complete Book of Shiatsu Therapy.*
4. Felix Mann, *Acupuncture, The Chinese Art of Healing and How It Works Scientifically,* p. 221.
5. Armand Lione, "Senility and Aluminum Poisoning," *Perspectives on Aging,* vol. X #d5, September/October, 1981, pp. 22–24.
6. Virginia Livingston-Wheeler and Edmond G. Addeo, *The Conquest of Cancer.*
7. Ibid., p. 173.
8. Ibid.
9. "Nutritional Individuality," *Journal of Nutritional Academy,* vol. 11 #11, pp. 13–23.

10. Cameron Stauth, "Supplement Boosts I.Q. in Retarded," *Medical News and International Reports*, vol. 5 #6, March 30, 1981, pp. 1, 6.

11. Letters to the Editor, *Sarasota Herald Tribune*, April 17, 1984, p. 5D.

12. Robert S. Mendelsohn, *Male Practice*, pp. 72–76.

13. Bob E. Jones, *The Difference a Doctor of Osteopathy Makes*.

14. Ann Hill, *Visual Encyclopedia of Unconventional Medicine*.

15. Marcus Bach, *The Chiropractic Story*.

16. Maesimund B. Panos, *Homeopathic Medicine at Home*.

17. Frederick LeBoyer, *Loving Hands*.

Glossary

This glossary provides definitions for words used in the text of this book and for terms you might encounter in your doctor's office.

ADRENAL GLANDS (ad-REEN-ul glandz)—triangular-shaped glands located near the upper surface of each kidney that produce adrenalin and cortisone.

AGAR (A-gar)—a kind of seaweed extracted and used primarily for bacterial culture media.

ALBUMIN (al-BU-min)—one of a group of simple proteins found in the blood, soluble in cold water, which coagulates with heat, then cannot be dissolved in cold or hot water. At times is found in the urine.

ALOPECIA (alo-PEE-sha)—loss of hair.

ALZHEIMER'S DISEASE (ALZ-hy-mer's disease)—a disease, of unknown cause, marked by a wasting away of parts of the brain. It usually attacks more women than men between the ages of forty and sixty.

ANDROGEN (AN-dro-jen)—a hormone responsible for the growth of male sex characteristics.

ANEMIA (a-NEE-mee-ya)—a condition in which the number of red blood cells is reduced. The anemic individual often will feel exhausted because the red cells are responsible for carrying oxygen through the body. Anemia is not a disease but may be a symptom of several possible diseases.

ANEROID (AN-er-oyd)—operating without a fluid, as in an aneroid barometer.

APLASTIC ANEMIA (a-PLAS-tik a-NEE-mee-ya)—an anemic condition in which the bone marrow makes an insufficient number of red blood cells.

ARTHRITIS (arth-RITE-us)—a disease which damages a joint or joints of the body, accompanied by varying degrees of inflammation and pain. Often involves distortion of the area.

AURICLES (AU-ri-culls)—the external part of the ear; also chambers of the heart.

BIBLIOGRAPHY (bib-lee-OG-ru-fee)—a list of books that presents title, author and publishing information.

BILE—fluid secreted by the liver, usually yellowish-brown or greenish in color, released to the upper part of the small intestine to mix with fats and aid digestion in the small intestine (duodenum).

BILIRUBIN (billy-ROO-bin)—the colored material in the bile carried to the liver by the blood and excreted into the urine and the stool.

BUERGER'S DISEASE (BURR-jer's disease)—a chronic disease which mainly affects the veins and arteries of the hands and feet.

CANKER (KANG-ker)—an open sore on the mouth or lips.

CARCINOMA (car-sin-OH-ma)—a cancerous tumor in the body.

CATARRH (cat-TAR)—inflammation of the mucous membranes usually resulting in a cough. An illness found more prevalently in the elderly.

CATHETER (KATH-e-ter)—a small hollow tube inserted to drain parts of the body where fluid has been retained.

CAT-SCRATCH DISEASE—an infection usually caused by a scratch from a diseased cat or an open cut exposed to a diseased cat. More prevalent in cooler weather, affecting children more than adults. Usually requires minor treatment.

CAUTERIZE (KAW-ter-ize)—use of heat, cold or chemicals to destroy harmful tissue.

CERVIX (SUR-vicks)—part of an organ that resembles a neck—e.g., the portion extending from the mouth of the uterus into the vagina is the *cervix uteri*.

CHANCRE (SHANG-kur)—a hard painless syphilitic primary ulcer which is the first sign of syphilis, appearing two to three weeks after eposure to the disease.

CHOLESTEROL (kul-ES-ter-ull)—a fat-soluble substance that occurs as an essential constituent of animal cells and body fluids. The substance has been implicated experimentally as a factor in arteriosclerosis. Animal tissues such as egg yolk and meat fats contain cholesterol and may contribute to high amounts of the substance in the body.

CHORIONIC GONADOTROPIN (KOR-ee-oh-nik gon-a-do-TRO-pin)—the hormone which becomes elevated during pregnancy. It is the substance measured by the pregnancy test.

CHRONIC (KRON-ik)—lasting a long time, showing little or no change over a long period of time.

COMA (COE-ma)—an unconscious state caused by illness or as a result of injury, often to the brain.

CONGESTION (kon-JES-chun)—too much blood or fluid in tissue or an organ of the body.

CONTAGIOUS (kon-TAY-jus)—transmitted easily from one person to another either directly or indirectly; *see* infectious.

CORTICOSTEROID (corti-COST-ter-oid)—hormonal steroid substance in the outer layer of the adrenal gland that speeds up biochemical reactions.

CULTURE (KULL-chur)—raising living tissue or organisms in material that encourages their growth, such as agar.

CYTOTOXIC AGENTS (sigh-toe-TOX-ik agents)—materials developed for use in chemotherapy, which are harmful to cells.

DEHYDRATION (DEE-hi-DRAY-shun)—when more water is taken out of a body or organ than is replaced.

DEPRESSED (dee-PREST)—a feeling of sadness and inability to do for oneself, inability to communicate, refusal to socialize.

DIABETES (dia-BEE-tus)—failure of the cells of the pancreas to secrete an adequate amount of insulin; characterized by frequency of urination, thirst and inability to produce sufficient insulin for the body's needs, which causes elevation of blood sugar. (Diabetes Insipidus is a disorder of the pituitary gland and has nothing to do with insulin production.)

DIAPHRAGM (DIA-fram)—a cup that fits over the cervix uteri and acts as a contraceptive, or the muscular wall separating the abdomen from the thoracic cavity which contracts and expands as you breathe.

DIASTOLE (DIA-stole)—part of the cycle during which the heart dilates and the cavity fills with blood.

DILATE (DI-late)—expand.

DIPSTICK (DIP-stick)—a strip of paper treated with chemicals and used for testing urine samples.

DIURETIC (die-yure-ET-ik)—an agent that increases the secretion of urine by increasing the flow of blood to the kidneys.

EDEMA (eh-DEEM-ah)—a condition of having large amounts of fluid in body tissues.

ELECTROCARDIOGRAM (ee-lek-tro-CAR-dee-o-gram)—a record tracing the electrical activity of the heart on a machine attached to the patient with wires.

EMBOLISM (EM-boh-lizm)—blockage either from a foreign substance or a blood clot that travels from one site to another and lodges in a blood vessel.

EMPHYSEMA (em-fy-SEEM-uh)—a condition that may be either temporary or chronic, characterized by air-filled expansions like blisters in the tissues of the lungs, or less commonly in other parts of the body. It could be caused by smoking, asthma, or air pollution, and gives rise to breathlessness, a husky cough, and frequently impairment of heart action.

ERYSIPELAS (era-SIP-a-lus)—contagious disease caused by a streptococcus infection with nausea, fever, red skin and sometimes blisters. Prognosis is good if treated promptly.

ETIOLOGY (ee-tee-OL-o-jy)—the science dealing with causes of disease.

FALSE NEGATIVE and FALSE POSITIVE—a reading at the end of a test that has given a result that is not correct. The false negative is an error that states you do not have a disease or illness, when further testing may show you do. The false positive error shows that you do have the disease or illness, when retesting shows you do not.

GANGRENE (gang-GREEN)—dead matter of the body resulting from lack of blood supply to the area.

GENERIC (jen-ER-ik)—a general term used to identify the original substance of medication. The generic form of a drug is often much cheaper than the brand-name medicine.

GLAUCOMA (glou-COE-ma)—an eye disease that shows up as pressure in the eyeball. If not treated, blindness may result.

GLOBULIN (GLOB-you-lin)—one of several kinds of simple proteins present in blood but not soluble in pure water.

GLUCOSE TOLERANCE TEST (GLU-cose tolerance test)—a test in which you swallow a measured amount of glucose, then have both urine and blood samples taken at stated intervals to determine your body's ability to metabolize glucose, and to diagnose diabetes or hypoglycemia.

GONADOTROPIN (go-nad-oh-TRO-pin)—a hormone that stimulates the gonads [male reproductive glands].

GOUT—a form of acute arthritis—perhaps a hereditary disease—noted for inflammation of the joints, usually the feet.

GYNECOLOGICAL (guy-ne-co-LOJ-i-cul)—pertaining to diseases affecting women.

HEPATITIS (hep-a-TIE-tus)—inflammation of the liver caused by infectious agents as well as certain drugs and poisons. Often accompanied by jaundice, liver enlargement and fever.

HEMOGLOBIN (HEEM-oh-glow-bin)—iron-containing pigment in the red blood cells that transports oxygen from the lungs to other parts of the body.

HOMEOSTASIS (home-ee-oh-STAY-sis)—equilibrium within the body maintained by a dynamic balance.

HYPERINSULINISM (hy-per-IN-su-lin-ism)—excessive amount of insulin in the blood which can cause hunger, weakness, sweating and double vision.

HYPERPITUITARISM (hy-per-pit-TOO-it-tare-ism)—overactivity of the pituitary glands in some middle-aged people resulting in elongation and enlargement of the bones of the hands and feet and even some head bones.

HYPOGLYCEMIA (hypo-gly-SEE-mee-ya)—deficiency of sugar in the blood causing acute fatigue, restlessness, malaise, weakness and irritability, fatigue or dizziness.

HYPOTHERMIA (hy-po-THERM-ee-ya)—a lower-than-normal body temperature. Sometimes produced artificially to facilitate surgical procedures. Due to less efficient circulation, older people must monitor their temperatures to avoid hypothermia.

HYPOTHYROIDISM (hy-po-THY-roid-ism)—underactivity of the thyroid gland, resulting in a lowered metabolic rate and loss of pep.

IATROGENIC DISORDER (EYE-a-tro-GEN-ik disorder)—an adverse mental or physical condition brought about as a result of medical treatment. The term implies that the condition could have been avoided with more judicious care.

INFECTIOUS (in-FEK-shus)—capable of transmitting disease due to the presence of a microorganism.

INTERNIST (in-TER-nist)—a physician who specializes in internal medicine.

IRIS (EYE-ris)—the round, colored part of the eye that frames the pupil and grows larger and smaller to regulate the amount of light entering the pupil.

KETONES (KEY-tones)—the end result of the digestion of fats; a simple ketone would be acetone.

LASSITUDE (LASS-i-tude)—tiredness, exhaustion.

LYMPH NODES (LIMF-nodes)—glands of varying size occurring singly or in groups, with blood vessels entering and leaving, carrying lymph to other parts of the body.

LYMPHOCYTE (LIM-fo-site)—white blood corpuscles that normally comprise 20 to 40 percent of the total of white blood cells. These may increase dramatically in leukemia or infection.

MAMMOGRAMS (MAM-oh-grams)—x-ray films for breast cancer.

METABOLISM (meh-TA-bo-lizm)—the total of all physical and chemical changes that take place in the body.

MONONEUCLEOSIS (MON-oh-noo-clee-OH-sis)—an infectious disease that affects the lymph nodes, spleen and often the liver. The illness shows up for four to seven weeks after exposure and is called the "kissing disease" because this is one of the ways it can be spread.

MYXEDEMA (mix-eh-DEE-ma)—underactivity of the thyroid gland, showing slow speech, dry skin and hair, sensitivity to cold, loss of mental and physical vigor.

NEURASTHENIA (noor-as-THEEN-ya)—a condition marked by exhaustion, depression, feelings of inadequacy and sometimes headache. There is often sensitivity to light and noise, poor digestion and circulation.

OMBUDSMAN (OM-boods-man)—a person, usually in the employ of the institution or hospital, who investigates reported complaints and helps to achieve equitable and satisfactory settlements. Also referred to as the "patient-advocate."

OPHTHALMOLOGIST (op-fthal-MOL-oh-gist)—a physician who specializes in the treatment of eye disorders.

OSTEOPOROSIS (os-tee-oh-paw-RO-sis)—a condition in which the skeleton has not been able to sustain normal functioning due to a calcium deficiency. Bones become thinner, weaker and more fragile, and break very easily. Most prevalent among elderly women.

PALPATE (PAL-pate)—the use of the hands and finger tips to examine the patient.

PAP SMEAR or *Papanicolaou Test*—collection of material from the cervix or vagina for microscopic study to help in diagnosing cancer.

PARATHYROID (par-a-THY-roid)—four small glands located at the lower edge of the thyroid gland. They secrete a hormone that regulates the body's use of calcium and phosphorus.

PERICARDIUM (per-ee-CARD-ee-yum)—the sac around the heart.

PETRI DISH (PEE-tree dish)—a shallow dish of plastic or glass with a cover, often prepared for use by the application of agar, for growing cultures in a laboratory.

PLACEBO (plah-SEE-bo)—a substance sometimes given to satisfy the patient's desire for medication. Also used in doing drug studies when some patients are given the medication to be tested and the others receive a sugar pill or *placebo*.

PROCTOSCOPY (proc-TOS-co-pee)—examination of the lower colon through the use of an instrument inserted into the rectum.

PROGNOSIS (prog-NO-sis)—an evaluation of the possible course or outcome of a disease or method of treatment.

PROSTATE (PROS-tate)—the gland that surrounds the neck of the bladder and the urethra in men.

PROTEIN (PRO-teen)—the basic component of body cells. Serves as a nitrogen source, aids in tissue building and is a source of energy. We derive proteins from the food we eat, especially cheese, eggs, fish, meat and milk. Proteins are digested in the stomach and pancreas and by bile salts produced in the liver. Infants, children, pregnant women and nursing mothers require extra protein in their diets.

PSYCHOSIS (sigh-COE-sis)—disintegration of the personality resulting in loss of contact with reality.

PUSTULES (PUS-tewls)—small blisters on the surface of the skin brought on by a variety of causes.

RENAL (REE-nul)—related to the kidney(s).

SIGMOID COLON (SIG-moid COE-lun)—the area of the colon that bends into the shape of the Greek letter "sigma", the ten inches of the gastrointestinal tract closest to the rectum.

SPECULUM (SPEC-you-lum)—instrument which opens wider a passage or body cavity to facilitate examination of an internal area of the body.

SPHYGMOMANOMETER (SFIG-mo-man-OM-e-ter)—an instrument for the measurement of blood pressure, described in chapter 1.

SPIROMETER (spy-RO-meeter)—instrument which measures inhalation and exhalation of breath.

SPONGY (SPUN-gy)—an area that is both porous and elastic.

STEROIDS (STEER-oids)—a group of compounds including some hormones, D vitamins, bile acids and certain sterols.

STETHOSCOPE (STETH-o-scope)—a y-shaped piece of rubber tubing, usually with a bell-like instrument at one end and tips to fit into the ears at the other, used to hear body sounds.

STREP THROAT (full name: streptococcus throat)—a sore throat caused by bacteria; often accompanied by fever and listlessness.

STRESS—a condition related to tension and strain, or any other situation in which there is a loss of equilibrium.

STUPOR (STOO-pur)—a state of unconsciousness.

SYSTEMIC DISEASE (sis-TEM-ic disease)—an illness that invades the whole body rather than one of its parts.

SYSTOLE (SIS-tole)—the contracting cycle of the heart, which forces the blood out toward the rest of the body. (*See* diastole.)

THERMOGRAPH (THERM-o-graf)—a diagnostic procedure for measuring the amount of heat in the body. Pictures can be made and saved for later reference. Sometimes used instead of the x-ray machine.

THYROGLOBULIN (thy-ro-GLOB-you-lin)—a protein that is iodine-containing.

THYROID GLAND (THY-roid gland)—located in front and on either side of the lower part of the larynx and upper part of the trachea. Gland produces thyroxine, which regulates body growth.

TRIGLYCERIDES (try-GLIH-ser-ides)—short chain fatty acids with glycerol. Most animal and vegetable fats are triglycerides.

TUMOR (TOO-mur)—a swelling forming an abnormal mass. Tumors are classified as benign (harmless) or malignant (cancerous). Different kinds of tumors can occur at various places on the body.

ULCER (UL-ser)—an infected cut or sore on the skin. Many kinds of ulcers may develop almost anywhere on the body.

URIC ACID (YOOR-ik acid)—a normal constituent of urine. This substance is implicated in gout, leukemia and other illnesses.

VDRL Test (full name: Venereal Disease Research Laboratory Test)—used in conjunction with pregnancy testing, marriage-license application blood testing, and testing for syphilis.

VEIN (vane)—a blood vessel that carries blood back to the heart and lungs, where it picks up oxygen.

VENTRICLE (VEN-trikle)—either of the two lower chambers of the heart.

VERTIGO (VER-tih-go)—a sensation of dizziness or giddiness as if one were moving around in space.

Select List of Organizations and Publications

Alcoholics Anonymous, National Office, 468 Park Avenue South, New York, NY 10016

Alzheimer's Disease and Related Disorders Association, 360 North Michigan Avenue, Suite 601, Chicago, IL 60601

American Academy of Family Physicians, 1740 West 2nd Street, Kansas City, MO 64114

American Aging Association, c/o Denham Harman, M.D., College of Medicine, University of Nebraska, Omaha, NB 68105. Write for information about data on latest advances in knowledge about aging.

American Cancer Society, 777 Third Avenue, New York, NY 10017. Information on checking for breast cancer and the progress of cancer research.

American Center for Homeopathy, 6560 Backlick Road, Suite 211, Springfield, VA 22150

American Chiropractic Association, 1916 Wilson Boulevard, Arlington, VA 22201

American Diabetes Association, Two Park Avenue, New York, NY 22314

American Foundation for Alternate Health Care, 25 Landfield Avenue, Monticello, NY 12701

American Geriatrics Society Inc., 10 Columbus Circle, Suite 1470, New York, NY 10019

American Group Practice Association, 1422 Duke Street, Alexandria, VA 22314.   Information about groups practicing in your area, either group specialists or multi-specialty groups.

American Heart Association, National Office, 7320 Greenville Avenue, Dallas, TX 75231

American Osteopathic Association, 212 East Ohio Street, Chicago, IL 60611

American Red Cross, 17th and D Streets N.W., Washington, DC 20006

Americans for Medical Freedom, 910 La Cresta Drive, Thousand Oaks, CA 91362

Arthritis Foundation, 1314 Spring Street N.W., Atlanta, GA 30309

Association for Medical and Health Alternatives, P.O. Box 112, Clearwater FL 33517

W.A. Baum Company, Copake, NY 11726

Boston Women's Health Book Collective, 465 Mount Auburn Street, Watertown, MA 02172

Coalition of Holistic Health Organizations, The, 1424 Sixteenth Street N.W., Suite 105, Washington, DC 20036

Consumer Information Center, Division of U.S. Government Printing Office, Dept. C, Pueblo, CO 81009

Dogs for the Deaf, 13260 Highway 238, Jacksonville, OR 97530

Harvard Community Health Plan, One Fenway Plaza, Boston, MA 02215.   Information about HMOs.

Health Insurance Plan of Greater New York, 220 West 58th Street, New York, NY 10022.   Information about HMOs.

International Association of Parents and Professionals for Safe Alternatives in Childbirth, P.O. Box 428, Marble Hill, MO 63764

International Institute of Reflexology, P.O. Box 12642, St. Petersburg, FL 33733

Johns Hopkins Hospital, 600 North Wolfe Street, Baltimore, MD 21205

Kaiser-Permanente Health Plan, 4747 Sunset Boulevard, Los Angeles, CA 90027

Living Bank, P.O. Box 6725, Houston, TX 77005.   To donate part or
all of your body on your death.
Medical Self-Care, P.O. Box 718, Inverness, CA 94937
Metropolitan Life Insurance Co., One Madison Avenue, New York,
NY 10017.   Information booklets on health available.
Midwives Alliance of North America, The Farm, Summertown, TN 38483
Mother Jones, 625 Third Street, San Francisco, CA 94103
National Burn Information Exchange, 200 North Ingalls, Ann Arbor, MI
48104
National Center for Homeopathy, 1500 Massachusetts Avenue NW, Suite
41, Washington, DC 20005.
National Herbalist Association, c/o International Institute for Biological
& Botanical Research, 271 Fifth Avenue, Suite 3, New York, NY
10016
National Women's Health Network, 224 Seventh Street SE, Washington,
DC 20003
Parkinson's Disease Foundation, William Black Medical Research Building,
Columbia Presbyterian Hospital, 640 West 168th Street, New York,
NY 10032
People's Doctor, P.O. Box 982, Evanston, IL 60204.   Newsletter published
by Dr. Robert B. Mendelsohn, author of several books debunking
some medical practices.
People's Medical Society,   14 East Minor Street, Emmaus, PA 18049
Physician's Desk Reference, Oradell, NJ 07649
Planned Parenthood Federation of America, National Office, 810
Seventh Avenue, New York, NY 10019
Sleep Research Society, c/o J. Christian Gillin, M.D., Dept. of Psychiatry,
University of California, La Jolla, CA 92093
Take Off Pounds Sensibly (TOPS), P.O. Box 07489, 4575 South 5th
Street, Milwaukee, WI 53207
United States Government Printing Office, North Cap Street, Washington,
DC 20402

Bibliography

Andrews, Lori B. *Deregulating Doctors*. Emmaus, PA: People's Medical
   Society, 1984.

Bach, Marcus. *The Chiropractic Story*. Los Angeles: De Vorss, 1968.

Bergson, Anika and Tuchak, Vladimir. *Shiatsu: The Japanese Pressure Point
   Massage*. Los Angeles: Pinnacle Books, 1976.

Bhaskar, S.N. *Synopsis of Oral Pathology*, 5th ed. St. Louis: Mosby Co., 1977.

Books in Print. New York: R. R. Bowker Co., 1983.

Boston Women's Health Collective. *Our Bodies, Ourselves*. New York: Simon
   & Schuster, 1979.

Chamberlain, E. Noble and Ogilvie, Colin M. *Symptoms and Signs in Clinical
   Medicine*. 9th edition. Chicago: Yearbook Publications, 1974.

Conn, Howard F., ed. *Current Therapy*. Philadelphia: W.B. Saunders Co.,
   1978.

Culbert, Michael L. *What The Medical Establishment Won't Tell You That Could
   Save Your Life*. Virginia Beach, VA: Donning Co. Publishers, 1983.

Cumulative Index Medicus. Bethesda, MD: National Library of Medicine, 1984.

Directory of Medical Specialists. Chicago: Marquis Who's Who Inc., 1984.

Dorland's Illustrated Medical Dictionary. Philadelphia: W.B. Saunders Co., 1980.

Dox, Ida; Melloni, John; and Eisner, Gilbert M. *Melloni's Illustrated Medical Dictionary.* Baltimore: Williams and Williams, 1979.

Dunlap, James. *Medical Negligence: The Uncontrolled Killer.* Miami, FL: World International Enterprises, 1977.

Gerras, Charles, ed. *The Complete Book of Vitamins.* Emmaus, PA: The Rodale Press, 1977.

Gibbons, Euell. *Stalking the Wild Asparagus.* New York: David McKay, Publishers, 1983.

Graedon, Joe. *The People's Pharmacy.* New York: St. Martin's Press, 1976.

Gupta, Yogi. *Yoga and Long Life.* New York: Dodd, Mead and Co., 1958.

Harley, Robison, D., ed. *Pediatric Ophthalmology.* Philadelphia: W.B. Saunders, 1983.

Harrison, Tinsley Randolph. *Harrison's Principles of Internal Medicine.* New York: McGraw-Hill, 1980.

Hittleman, Richard. *Richard Hittleman's Introduction to Yoga.* New York: Bantam Books, 1969.

How Your Blood Pressure is Measured. Copake, New York: W.A. Baum Co., Inc.

Illich, Ivan. *Medical Nemesis: The Expropriation of Health.* New York: Pantheon Books, 1982.

Index Medicus. Bethesda, MD: National Library of Medicine, 1984.

Jonas, Steven. *Medical Mystery: The Training of Doctors in the United States.* New York: W. W. Norton, 1978.

Jones, Bob. *The Difference a Doctor of Osteopathy Makes.* Oklahoma City, OK: Times-Journal Publishing Co., 1978.

Kirschmann, John D. *Nutrition Almanac, Revised Edition.* New York: McGraw-Hill Book Co., 1979.

Knowles, John H., ed. *Doing Better and Feeling Worse: Health in the United States.* New York: W.W. Norton Co., 1977.

Kra, Siegfried J. *Examine Your Doctor: A Patient's Guide to Avoiding Medical Mishaps.* New Haven, CT: Ticknor and Fields, 1982.

Krieger, Dolores. *The Therapeutic Touch.* Englewood Cliffs, NJ: Prentice-Hall, 1979.

Krupp, Marcus A. and Chatton, Milton J., ed. *Current Medical Diagnosis and Treatment.* Los Altos, CA: Lange Medical Publishers, 1982.

LeBoyer, Frederick. *Loving Hands*. New York: Alfred A. Knopf, 1976.

Livingston-Wheeler, Virginia and Addeo, Edmond G. *The Conquest of Cancer*. New York: Franklin Watts, Publishers, 1984.

Mann, Felix. *Acupuncture: The Ancient Chinese Art of Healing and How It Works Scientifically*. New York: Vintage Press, 1973.

Medical Self-Care., Inverness, CA.

Medical Books in Print. New York: R.R. Bowker, Co., 1983.

Mendelsohn, Robert S. *Confessions of a Medical Heretic*. New York: Warner Books, 1979.

_____. *Male Practice: How Doctors Manipulate Women*. Chicago: Contemporary Books, 1982.

Mother Jones, San Francisco, CA, Foundation for National Progress. Journal published nine times/year.

Namikoshi, Toru. *The Complete Book of Shiatsu Therapy*. San Francisco: Japanese Trading Co., 1980.

Oxford English Dictionary. New York: Oxford University Press, 1982.

Panos, Maesimund B. *Homeopathic Medicine at Home*. Los Angeles: J. P. Tarcher, Publishers, 1980.

Physician's Desk Reference. Oradell, NJ: Medical Economics Books, 1983.

Pinckney, Cathey and Pinckney, Edward R. *Do-It-Yourself Medical Testing: More Than 160 Tests You Can Do At Home*. New York: Facts-on-File Publications, 1983.

_____. *The Encyclopedia of Medical Tests*. New York: Facts-on-File Publications, 1982.

_____. *The Patient's Guide to Medical Tests*. New York: Facts-on-File Publications, 1982.

Riggs, Carol. *Herbs, Leaves of Magic*. Boulder, CO: Sycamore Island Books, 1979.

Rosenfeld, Isadore. *The Complete Medical Examination*. New York: Simon & Schuster, 1978.

_____. *Second Opinion*. New York: Simon & Schuster, 1981.

Satchadananda, Yogiraj Sri Swami. *Integral Yoga Hatha*. New York: Holt, Rinehart and Winston, 1970.

Schaefer, R.C., ed. *Chiropractic Health Care: A Conservative Approach to Health Restoration, Maintenance, and Disease Resistance*. Des Moines, IA: The Foundation for Chiropractic Education and Research, 1977.

Sehnert, Keith W. and Eisenberg, Howard. *How To Be Your Own Doctor— Sometimes*. New York: Grosset and Dunlap, 1975.

Silverman, Harold M. and Simon, Gilbert I. *The Pill Book*. New York: Bantam Books, 1979.

Taber's Cyclopedic Dictionary. Philadelphia: F.A. Davis Co., 1981.

Toguchi, Masaru. *The Complete Guide to Acupuncture*. New York: Frederick Fell, Publishers, 1974.

Visual Encyclopedia of Unconventional Medicine. Edited by Ann Hill. New York: Crown Publishing Co., 1978.

Wasco, James. *Not For Doctors Only*. Reading, MA: Addison-Wesley, 1980.

Wolfe, Sidney M. *Pills That Don't Work*. Washington, DC: D.C. Health Research Group Publications, 1980.

Index

Annette Thornhill

Annette Thornhill is a former medical librarian and teacher, and holds a master's degree from the University of Connecticut. She created and ran the medical library at Fairfield Hills Hospital in Newtown, Connecticut, and was a trustee for the self-help program at Connecticut College.

Since her retirement, Ms. Thornhill has dedicated herself to improving the quality of health care, especially for the elderly, and to making sure the providers of medical care are responsible and accountable to their patients. She is the health committee chairperson for the Sarasota, Florida chapter of the Gray Panthers and was a representative for the Florida Silver-Haired Legislature in 1985. She also established the Sarasota chapter of the People's Medical Society. A tireless consumer advocate, Ms. Thornhill is a registered lobbyist in the state of Florida for the health care field and has appeared before the Florida Senate and House of Representatives on such issues as health statutes, patients' rights, and medical malpractice.

Ms. Thornhill's active retirement includes traveling throughout the United States in her personal motor home with her dog. She is a living example of her teachings, and places great value on proper nutrition, exercise, a positive mental attitude, and personal involvement in maintaining good health.